Parasitology

Symposia of the British Society for Parasitology Volume 38

Parasite variation: immunological and ecological significance

EDITED BY
MARK E. VINEY and ANDREW F. READ

CO-ORDINATING EDITOR
L. H. CHAPPELL

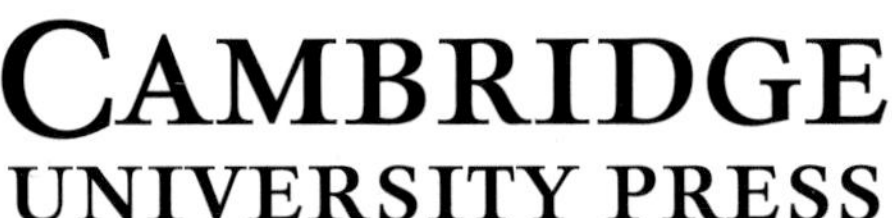
CAMBRIDGE
UNIVERSITY PRESS

Contents

List of contributions

Symposia of the British Society for Parasitology
VOLUME 38

Parasite variation: immunological and ecological significance

EDITED BY MARK VINEY AND ANDREW READ

CO-ORDINATING EDITOR L. H. CHAPPELL

Preface

All organisms vary genetically and, hence, phenotypically. This variation is the stuff of evolution. This variation also affects where organisms live and what they can do to each other and to their environment. In these respects, micro- and macro-parasites are no different than any other organisms. The only special condition is that a significant part of their habitat is other organisms. Parasite variation which alters the interaction with the host environment should be of particular anthropocentric interest and significance. Variation that brings about reduced host fitness means disease and increased host mortality; variation that increases host fitness is a means by which we can effect parasite control.

Yet, with a few notable exceptions, parasitologists have not had a glorious history of taking account of virtually any aspect of parasite variation. Much parasitology is based on a single, long-term laboratory isolate maintained in a host (= environment) in which it does not naturally occur. This is true even for many of the protozoa, where there is overwhelming evidence of substantial genetic variation. It is hugely unlikely that this variation has no implications for our understanding of pathogenesis, infection and transmission. A paradox for sociologists of science is why it is that parasitologists typically ignore phenotypic variation in traits that matter, while geneticists have a long and noble history of investigating some of the least important traits imaginable (e.g. number of bristles on a *Drosophila* leg).

Parasites of vertebrates have to contend with the acquired immune response, an adaptive, dynamic and potentially deadly host defence. Given the huge selection pressure this must impose on parasites, determining how parasites deal with immunity is to not only understand a remarkable aspect of biology, but also something of practical significance. Yet, here it is hard not to feel that the forest is being lost for the trees. We have an ever more exquisite understanding of the molecular control of antigenic variation in some taxa (e.g. trypanosomes) and are racing towards the same goal in others (e.g. *Plasmodium*). Conventional wisdom posits that antigenic variation has evolved for immune evasion, but there is no direct evidence to show that antigenic variation actually increases parasite transmission. It may be difficult to understand why else it exists, and the fact that so much genome is given over to it certainly argues that it must have some important fitness consequences. But we should not accept something just because we lack the imagination to consider alternatives. Moreover, if the idea is right, it ought to be able to explain why, for instance, an antigen repertoire is not larger or smaller. Further, we should not overlook challenging data: the free-living ciliate *Paramecium* has antigenic variation too, yet they never encounter a vertebrate immune system.

Parasite variation may also be responsible for variation in disease severity. Despite the many studies trying to find host genes associated with the outcome of parasite disease, we know of only one which has attempted to estimate just how important host genetic variation really is (Mackinnon *et al.* 2000). In that case, it explained about 10% of the variance in disease severity, even though the study concerned malaria parasites, one of the textbook situations where host genes are supposed to be important. Measured environmental variables accounted for perhaps another

Parasitology (2002), **125**, S1–S2.
DOI: 10.1017/S0031182002002500 Printed in the United Kingdom

20% of the variation, but what explains the remaining variation? Surely it is time to measure the contribution of parasite variation to disease severity?

The papers in this volume are the result of a meeting that considered parasite variation with a particular focus on its environmental significance. The full range of parasites were represented, and were considered from an empirical, theoretical (and even anecdotal) view. It is clear that there is substantial variation within and between genotypes of parasitic protozoa, but that the actual effect of this in infections is still unclear. It is also abundantly clear that helminths vary in very many important ways, if one bothers to look. What does all this variation mean?

A recurring theme of the talks, and the papers in this volume, is the difficulty of obtaining relevant experimental data about the ecological and immunological significance of parasite variation. Endoparasite variation is hard to work with, even where appropriate animal models exist. Many of the phenotypes are ephemeral, and many depend on the precise environment in which the parasites are present. And while numerous laboratories have worked on a diversity of rodent hosts, because they can be readily obtained, almost all work with a single parasite strain. Part of this is surely habit, but it is difficult to escape the feeling that focusing on parasite variation is to open a can of worms. If we allow that host variation, parasite variation, the environment *and* the two-way and the three-way interactions are all important determinants of disease and epidemiology, we need vast numbers of experimental treatments to make progress. Nonetheless, ignoring complexities is not the way to understand them.

The meeting took place in London at the Linnean Society of London only yards from the building where Darwin and Wallace presented their joint paper on the significance of biological variation. We thank the Society for their outstanding hospitality, particularly their enthusiastic distribution of wine. The meeting took place three days after the 11th September terrorists attacks. The resulting chaos prevented Dennis Minchella (Purdue University, IN, USA) from presenting the Wellcome Trust lecture. We are grateful nevertheless for his contribution to this volume. Two of the talks given on the day do not appear in this volume: Andrew Read filled Prof. Minchella's programme slot with a talk about virulence variation in malaria parasites, and Chris Newbold gave a stimulating view of antigenic variation in *Plasmodium*. We are grateful to all the contributors for their contributions to the meeting and this volume, and to Les Chappell and John Lewis for gentle and not so gentle nudges at usually appropriate times. We are grateful to the Wellcome Trust and Cambridge University Press for financial support for the meeting.

REFERENCES

MACKINNON, M. J., GUNAWARDENA, D. M., RAJAKARUNA, J., WEERASINGHA, S., MENDIS, K. N. & CARTER, R. (2000). Quantifying genetic and nongenetic contributions to malarial infection in a Sri Lankan population. *Proceedings of the National Academy of Sciences, USA* **97**, 12661–12666.

Measuring immune selection

D. J. CONWAY* *and* S. D. POLLEY

Department of Infectious and Tropical Diseases, London School of Hygiene and Tropical Medicine, Keppel St, London WC1E 7HT

SUMMARY

Immune responses that kill pathogens or reduce their reproductive rate are generally important in protecting hosts from infection and disease. Pathogens that escape the full impact of such responses will survive, and any heritable genetic basis of this evasion will be selected. Due to the memory component of vertebrate immune responses, pathogens with rare alleles of a target antigen can have an advantage over those with common alleles, leading to the maintenance of a polymorphism. At the genetic level, there ought to be detectable signatures of balancing selection in the genes encoding these antigens. Here, methods for identifying these selective signatures are reviewed. Their practical utility for identifying which antigens are targets of protective immune responses is discussed.

Key words: Antigens, genes, protective immunity, natural selection, tests of neutrality.

INTRODUCTION

Immune responses to pathogens involve diverse mechanisms, directed against many different target epitopes. However, only a minority of these responses may be protective to the host. Empirical description of all immune responses in natural infections is an enormous task which is not guaranteed to identify the protective responses. Methods for focusing research efforts on protective immune responses are therefore desirable.

Logically, mechanisms and targets of protective immunity should be best understood in studies of pathogens with small genomes and few expressed proteins. The specificity of responses to particular viruses, including Human Immunodeficiency Virus-1 (HIV-1) and related viruses in monkeys has been dissected in fine detail. Concurrent study of genetic variation in the hosts and in the viruses has proved critical in understanding which responses are protective (Evans *et al.* 1999; Allen *et al.* 2000; Kelleher *et al.* 2001). There is tight genetic restriction of cytotoxic T cell (CTL) responses against viral peptides, with differences between hosts in MHC class I alleles determining whether an effective response is made. Due to the high viral mutation rate, mutants with alterations in CTL epitope sequences frequently arise, and their growth and selection is affected by the specificity of the CTL response in the host (Goulder *et al.* 2001). It has even been noted that where selection of sequence variants is not seen, this is evidence for the absence of a protective immune response to that sequence (Hay *et al.* 1999). This may be an extreme system, but it raises the question of whether an understanding of immune selection on pathogen antigens may be generally useful.

* Corresponding author: Tel: +44 (0)20 7927 2331. Fax: +44 (0)20 7636 8739. E-mail: david.conway@lshtm.ac.uk

POLYMORPHIC AND VARIANT ANTIGENS

It is observed that many pathogen antigens are polymorphic (multiple allelic forms existing in the species), and many others undergo variation within a clone (due to the differential expression of multiple loci in the genome). Examples of single-locus antigen genes that are highly polymorphic in pathogens of humans or domestic animals are given in Table 1, and examples of multi-locus genes responsible for antigenic variation are given in Table 2. The significance of such polymorphism and variation is not known in most cases. Particular protein domains may be involved in pathogen adhesion to (or invasion of) host cells, causing variation in tissue tropism and virulence. Additionally, these or other domains may be targets of protective immune responses. The distribution and function of polymorphism and variation therefore warrants investigation.

The range of pathogens with single-locus polymorphic (Table 1) and multi-locus variant (Table 2) antigens is very similar. The one obvious exception is that viruses with small genomes cannot have multi-locus antigen genes, but otherwise the existence of either polymorphic or variant antigens appears not to be phylogenetically restricted. Virtually all of the polymorphic or variant antigens known so far have a surface location. It may also be noted that the majority of polymorphic antigens (Table 1) are on the invasive stages of the pathogens, whereas most of the variant antigens (Table 2) are on the surface of infected cells or on extracellular pathogens. This latter trend is not absolute, and there is at least one example known of a variant

Parasitology (2002), **125**, S3–S16. © 2002 Cambridge University Press
DOI: 10.1017/S0031182002002214 Printed in the United Kingdom

Table 1. Examples of highly polymorphic single-locus antigen genes in major pathogens of humans or domestic animals

Pathogen	Gene	Location of protein	Reference[a]
HIV-1	*env*	Surface of invasive virus	(Vidal *et al.* 2000)
Influenza A	*H*	Surface of invasive virus	(Tsuchiya *et al.* 2001)
Chlamydia trachomatis	*omp1*	Surface of invasive stage	(Stothard *et al.* 1998)
Neisseria gonorrhoeae	*por*	Porin in bacterial membrane	(Fudyk *et al.* 1999)
Borrelia burgdorferi	*ospA*	Surface of pathogen	(Rannala *et al.* 2000)
	ospC	Surface of pathogen	(Rannala *et al.* 2000)
Theileria annulata	*Tams1*	Surface of invasive merozoite	(Gubbels *et al.* 2000)
Babesia bovis	*msa-1*	Surface of invasive merozoite	(Suarez *et al.* 2000)
Plasmodium falciparum	*msp1*	Surface of invasive merozoite	(Miller *et al.* 1993)
	msp2	Surface of invasive merozoite	(Felger *et al.* 1997)
	msp3	Merozoite surface associated	(McColl & Anders, 1997)
	ama1	Apical rhopteries of merozoite	(Verra & Hughes, 1999)
	S-antigen	Secreted	(Anderson & Day, 2000)

[a] References are examples which analyse the gene polymorphisms, but are not necessarily primary descriptions. Original characterization of the genes, data on the structures and putative functions of the proteins they encode and further information on polymorphism may be found in other papers cited in these references.

Table 2. Examples of multi-locus genes encoding variant antigens in major pathogens of humans or domestic animals

Pathogen	Gene	Location of protein	Reference[a]
Anaplasma marginale	*msp1b*	Surface of pathogen	(Viseshakul *et al.* 2000)
	msp2	Surface of pathogen	(Brayton *et al.* 2001)
	msp3	Surface of pathogen	(Brayton *et al.* 2001)
Borrelia burgdorferi	*vlsE*	Surface of pathogen	(Zhang & Norris, 1998)
Chlamydia trachomatis	*pmp*	Outer membrane of pathogen	(Stephens & Lammel, 2001)
Neisseria gonorrhoeae	*pilE*	Pilus on surface of pathogen	(Mehr *et al.* 2000)
Pneumocystis carinii	*msg*	Surface of pathogen	(Stringer & Keely, 2001)
Babesia bovis	*ves1a*	Infected erythrocyte surface	(Allred *et al.* 2000)
Plasmodium falciparum	*var*	Infected erythrocyte surface	(Smith *et al.* 2001)
Trypanosoma brucei	*vsg*	Surface of pathogen	(Borst & Ulbert, 2001)

[a] References are examples that include recent results and give an overview of each system. Primary descriptions and many earlier studies are cited within these.

antigen expressed in an invasive stage of a rodent malaria parasite (Preiser *et al.* 1999), but it may be worth future attention.

A common hypothesis is that there is frequency-dependent selection on antigens, so that a pathogen with a rare antigenic type is more likely to escape acquired immune responses than a pathogen with a common type. This depends on the memory component of vertebrate immune responses, and the advantage of the rare type is soon lost if it becomes very common. In the case of polymorphic antigens encoded by single gene loci in the pathogen genome (Fig. 1A), this would be an effective means of selection maintaining different alleles within populations. This would not indicate that the pathogen has a 'strategy' to escape immune responses, but rather the opposite. It is simply the result of ongoing allele-specific mortality of the pathogen, from which no allele has found an escape to fixation.

Antigens encoded by multiple variant gene loci can provide another means of survival, as a single pathogen clone has a range of options for expression (Fig. 1B). The genetic mechanisms by which phenotypic switching occurs within a clone will affect the type of selection to which the pathogen is subjected. In a single clone infection, antigenic phenotypes may switch without any changes occurring in the genome, by alteration of gene transcription. Immune selection among the various phenotypes will not lead to heritable change in a population of identical clones. However, selection may occur between genotypically different pathogens, and this selection would potentially involve the whole repertoire of gene loci encoding the variant antigens (together with the switching mechanism itself).

So, why do polymorphic single-locus antigen genes under balancing selection not always evolve into multi-locus genes by duplication? It would seem to be generally advantageous for a pathogen genome to contain options for many antigenic types and to temporally express different alternative rare types,

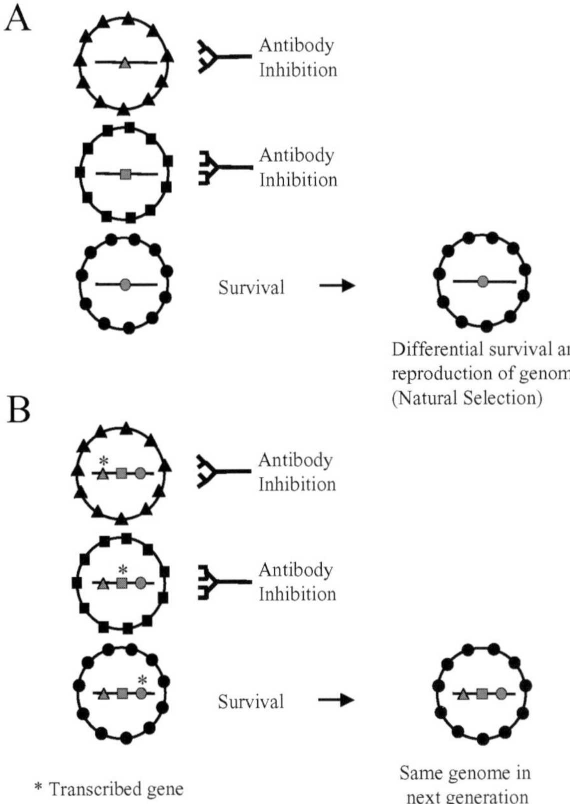

Fig. 1. A. Scheme of immune selection on a polymorphic pathogen surface antigen (3 different clones within a host). Allele-specific immune responses cause differential survival of the unrecognised genotype, and thus natural selection on heritable variation. B. Scheme of immune selection on transcriptionally-determined phenotypes of a variant pathogen surface antigen encoded by 3 variant genes (with 3 different phenotypes of one clone within a host). Variant-specific immune responses cause differential survival of the unrecognised phenotype, but this has an identical genotype to the other variants so there is no heritable change.

rather than encoding and expressing only one type that is subject to greater mortality when common. However, the existence of a highly effective and exclusive expression switching mechanism would be a logical pre-requisite for a hypothetical selective advantage of antigen gene duplication and diversification in the genome. A pathogen with an increased antigenic repertoire, which was constantly expressed, would be likely to have a serious disadvantage. It would thus appear that evolution of multi-locus systems of antigenic variation requires co-evolution of the antigenic repertoire (due to duplication and changes in the antigen gene coding sequences) and the regulation of their expression (due to changes in the promoter sequences and the expression of transcription factors which bind to them, or possibly involving other mechanisms). This requirement for co-evolution of repertoire and regulation could be a general impediment to the evolution of antigen variation systems.

Here, a simple question is considered which is relevant to either single-locus or multi-locus systems. How is it possible to identify which antigens are under selection by immune responses, and moreover, to identify the particular domains under the strongest selection?

SIGNATURES OF SELECTION ON ANTIGEN GENES

An understanding of selection on multi-locus variant antigen genes will be highly complex. The heritability of a switch in antigenicity may be uncertain, and not necessarily determined by whether there is a change at the DNA sequence level. Some transcriptional changes result from 'epigenetic' modification of parts of the genome, for example by methylation of DNA or acetylation of histones, at specific loci or whole chromosomal regions such as telomeres. These modifications may affect the phenotypes of subsequent generations, and in that sense display a form of inheritance. In eukaryotes, the existence and mechanisms of epigenetic inheritance differs among phylogenetic groups (Martienssen & Colot, 2001), and it is likely that they differ greatly among pathogens. Conversely, some mutational changes in DNA sequences are inherently unstable and may not be heritable in the long-term. In particular, homopolymeric tracts (continuous runs of a single nucleotide) are liable to a high frequency of slip-strand mutation leading to the loss or gain of a single nucleotide, leading to frameshifts within coding sequences (Parkhill *et al.* 2000). This provides a mechanism of 'phase variation' which switches protein expression on and off in different generations, and therefore is potentially important in varying the expression of antigens and other virulence genes. For each system of antigen variation, thorough genomic and transcriptional characterization of the genes is ideally required as a basis for studies of natural selection.

In contrast, testing for signatures of selection on single-locus genes can be relatively straightforward, at least in principle. This is because of the development of the neutral theory of molecular evolution (Kimura, 1983; Li, 1997). Understanding how genes will vary and diverge in populations without selection (due to mutation, gene frequency drift, population division, and migration), and how they are constrained by negative selection on deleterious mutations, provides a means of noting the exceptions (i.e. genes at which the polymorphism is influenced by positive selection). A common misconception is that genetic variation that shows a non-random pattern is evidence of selection. In fact, neutral processes do not normally lead to random patterns in DNA variation, but rather to a range of possible patterns, caused by the combined effects of mutation, recombination, gene frequency drift, and population size and structure. The expected range of neutral variation can only be predicted by a consideration of the processes themselves. There is extensive statistical understanding of the patterns of nucleotide variation that can occur under neutrality, allowing expectations to be made under different models, and thereby allowing the detection of significant observed departures from these (Kreitman, 2000).

METHODS FOR DETECTING SELECTION ON GENES

It is of practical importance to consider which of these analytical methods are most useful for detecting evidence of selection on pathogen antigen genes. One way in which this may be approached is to compare the results of previous studies. It is of particular interest to examine a number of different statistical tests applied to the same antigen gene, or alternatively to examine the results of the same test applied to different antigen genes. The malaria parasite *Plasmodium falciparum* has the largest number of polymorphic single-locus antigen genes yet described, of which 13 have been explored for evidence of selection by one method or another, which should provide a reasonably broad base for such preliminary comparisons. These are listed in Table 3 (with criteria for inclusion given in the footnote). Four of the methods listed, named after their inventors (Watterson, 1978; Tajima, 1989; McDonald & Kreitman, 1991; Fu & Li, 1993), are formal tests of whether patterns of polymorphism in a given locus depart from neutral expectations. The remaining two, dN/dS ratio and fixation (F_{ST}) indices, are effective for comparative analyses of variation in multiple genes or regions of a gene, to detect loci which are unusual (Nei & Gojobori, 1986; McDonald, 1994). The dN/dS ratio, i.e. the ratio of the proportion of nonsynonymous (amino-acid altering) nucleotide allelic differences per nonsynonymous site versus the proportion of synonymous (silent) differences per synonymous site, can also operate in principle as a formal test of neutrality. However, this is skewed by biases in nucleotide composition and codon usage in many organisms, including *P. falciparum*, so other approaches to account for this are required.

In Table 3, the *P. falciparum* antigen genes marked with an asterisk for a given analysis show where data were indicative of diversifying selection. Evidence of selection on the *ama1* gene (encoding apical membrane antigen 1 in the micronemes of the invasive merozoite stage) has emerged from all four different approaches applied to it (McDonald-Kreitman, dN/dS ratio, Tajima's, and Fu & Li's tests). Similarly, there are indications of selection from each of the three analyses applied to *msp2* (dN/dS ratio, Ewens-Watterson, and F_{ST}), the two analyses applied to *glurp* (McDonald-Kreitman, and Ewens-Watterson), the two analyses applied to *pfs48/45* (McDonald-Kreitman, and F_{ST}), and the two analyses applied to *lsa-1* (McDonald-Kreitman, and dN/dS ratio). Conversely, there was no evidence of selection from either of two analyses of the *S-antigen* gene (dN/dS ratio, and F_{ST}) or two analyses of the *pfs25* gene (McDonald-Kreitman, and dN/dS ratio). For all of the above genes, the different analyses lead to very concordant results. From this, it is reasonable to conclude that there is stronger evidence of selection on the *ama1*, *msp2*, *glurp*, *lsa-1*, and *pfs48/45* genes than on the *S-antigen* or *pfs25* genes.

For some other antigen genes (e.g. *csp*, *msp1*, and *eba-175*) there are apparent differences between analyses in Table 3, with evidence of selection provided by one test but not another. It is these latter cases that might be expected to discriminate between tests (regarding their power or validity). Do some tests yield false positive results, or are other tests inherently lacking in power? It is not clear that either problem exists, because of the different nature and size of the data sets analysed by each of the tests, meaning that accurate comparison between tests cannot be done. Moreover, different regions of the *msp1* and *eba-175* genes were studied in the different tests applied to each gene, so the results are not comparable. In summary, it is advisable to employ multiple analyses in the investigation of evidence of selection on a gene. Most tests are informative to some extent, and it is not clear from Table 3 whether any one test has generally proved more useful than others. However, the amount and the nature of the data needed for each type of analysis differs, and this may prove the deciding factor for future work which is likely to require study of larger numbers of genes. The sequence-based method which probably requires fewest samples and the least amount of sequencing is the McDonald-Kreitman test.

A CLOSE EXAMINATION OF ONE METHOD

We will consider the performance of the McDonald-Kreitman test in more detail. Table 4 shows the results of this test applied to 9 different antigen genes of *P. falciparum*. This test examines the numbers of polymorphic nucleotides which are synonymous (silent) and non-synonymous (amino acid altering), in a sample of *P. falciparum* alleles, and also the number of synonymous and non-synonymous nucleotide fixed differences between *P. falciparum* and the homologous gene from a closely-related species (in this case the chimpanzee parasite *P. reichenowi*). At each level, intra-specific and inter-specific, it is observable that there are more non-synonymous than synonymous differences. This observation in itself may be expected in the absence of any positive or negative selection. This is firstly because of the trivial but universal feature that most nucleotide

Table 3. Molecular population genetic studies testing for evidence of selection on *P. falciparum* polymorphic antigen genes

Method	Data used	Gene	Reference
McDonald-Kreitman	DNA sequences of alleles and a closely-related species	*csp*	(Escalante *et al.* 1998)
		*lsa-1**	(Escalante *et al.* 1998)
		rap-1	(Escalante *et al.* 1998)
		*pfs48/45**	(Escalante *et al.* 1998)
		pfs25	(Escalante *et al.* 1998)
		*ama1**	(Kocken *et al.* 2000; Polley & Conway, 2001)
		*eba-175**	(Ozwara *et al.* 2001)
		msp3	(Okenu *et al.* 2000)
		*glurp**	(Theisen *et al.* 2001)
dN/dS ratio	DNA sequences of alleles	*csp**	(Hughes & Hughes, 1995; Escalante *et al.* 1998)
		*lsa-1**	(Escalante *et al.* 1998)
		*trap**	(Hughes & Hughes, 1995)
		msp1	(Escalante *et al.* 1998)
		*msp2**	(Hughes & Hughes; 1995; Escalante *et al.* 1998)
		*msp3**	(Escalante *et al.* 1998)
		*ama1**	(Verra & Hughes, 1999)
		pfs25	(Hughes & Hughes, 1995)
		S-antigen	(Hughes & Hughes, 1995; Anderson & Day, 2000)
Tajima's D	DNA sequences of randomly sampled alleles from one population	*ama1**	(Polley & Conway, 2001)
Fu & Li's D & F	DNA sequences of randomly sampled alleles from one population	*ama1**	(Polley & Conway, 2001)
Ewens-Watterson	Randomly sampled alleles from one population	*msp1*	(Conway, 1997)
		*msp2**	(Conway, 1997)
		*glurp**	(Conway, 1997)
Fixation indices (F_{ST})	Allele frequencies in different populations	*msp1**	(Conway *et al.* 2000*a*)
		*msp2**	(Conway, 1997; Hoffman *et al.* 2001)
		eba-175	(Binks *et al.* 2001)
		*pfs48/45**	(Conway *et al.* 2001)
		S-antigen	(Anderson & Day, 2000)

An asterisk (*) indicates where results led to an inference of diversifying selection on a particular gene. Studies are included if they analysed at least the following minimal amount of sampled data for each test: McDonald-Kreitman test, 5 alleles of *P. falciparum* and 1 sequence of *P. reichenowi*; dN/dS ratio, 10 alleles of *P. falciparum*; Tajima's and Fu & Li's tests, 20 alleles of *P. falciparum* randomly sampled from a population; Ewens-Watterson test, 100 alleles of *P. falciparum* randomly sampled from a population.

positions in coding sequences are non-synonymous (synonymous positions are mainly at the third position in codons). Secondly, in the case of *Plasmodium* there is a particularly restricted codon usage (some synonymous alternative codons being scarcely used) due to the extreme A+T richness of the genome. However, as these general effects are the same for both *P. falciparum* and *P. reichenowi* (which have similar codon usage), bias will not affect the McDonald-Kreitman test here (but care needs to be taken when applying this test to other species). For this procedure, to test whether non-synonymous or synonymous differences are particularly skewed in ratios within a species or between species, a 2×2 table is constructed. Fisher's exact test of significance is applied, and the 'Neutrality Index' odds ratio shows to what extent there is an excess (odds ratio > 1) or deficit (< 1) of within-species nonsynonymous polymorphisms.

Five of the nine genes analysed in Table 4 show a significant excess of intra-specific non-synonymous versus synonymous polymorphism (compared to the ratios for inter-specific differences), including genes encoding antigens considered prime candidates for a blood-stage malaria vaccine (*ama1*, *eba-175*, *glurp*). The significant results do not simply go with the genes which have a lot of sequence polymorphism. The results are rather more revealing, possibly even surprising. The most highly significant result is for *lsa-1* (the gene encoding liver stage antigen-1),

Table 4. Neutrality index and significance of the McDonald-Kreitman test for nucleotide polymorphism in *P. falciparum* antigen genes compared with divergence from their *P. reichenowi* homologues

Gene	Intraspecific (*P.f.*) Syn	Intraspecific (*P.f.*) Nsyn	Interspecific (*P.f. vs P.r.*) Syn	Interspecific (*P.f. vs P.r.*) Nsyn	Neutrality Index Odds Ratio[a] (with 95% CI)	*P* value[b]	Reference[c]
csp	4	20	4	34	0·6 (0·1–3·6)	n.s.	(Escalante *et al.* 1998)
lsa-1	0	16	15	25	∞ (undefined)	0·003	(Escalante *et al.* 1998)
rap-1	0	7	16	48	∞ (undefined)	n.s.	(Escalante *et al.* 1998)
ama1	9	56	18	40	2·8 (1·1–7·6)	0·02	(Kocken *et al.* 2000)
msp3	22	70	0	10	0·0 (0·0–1·56)	n.s.	(Okenu *et al.* 2000)
eba-175	1	16	47	114	6·6 (1·0–282·4)	0·044	(Ozwara *et al.* 2001)
glurp	2	19	17	32	5·1 (1·0–48·9)	0·04	(Theisen *et al.* 2001)
pfs48/45	0	6	13	12	∞ (undefined)	0·03	(Escalante *et al.* 1998)
pfs25	5	7	10	15	0·9 (0·2 – 4·9)	n.s.	(Escalante *et al.* 1998)

[a] Odds for likelihood of a nonsynonymous difference to be polymorphic within *P. falciparum* rather than different between the species.
[b] *P* value from Fisher's exact test. n.s., not significant.
[c] References and data are from the first published use of the McDonald-Kreitman test on each given gene.

indicating strong diversifying selection on the amino acid sequence in *P. falciparum*. LSA-1 has been previously noted to have few amino acid polymorphisms, encouraging hopes that a vaccine might be based on conserved sequences in this case (Fidock *et al.* 1994; Aidoo *et al.* 1995). However, what matters here (and everywhere else) is the quality rather than the quantity of allelic differences. For example, at position 85 in the LSA-1 protein there are 3 amino acid alleles, due to 3 different nucleotides at the first position in the codon (highly unlikely under neutrality given the low overall polymorphism). Interestingly, synthetic peptides including the alternatives at this position have very different binding profiles to human HLA class I alleles, and interferon γ responses (putatively by cytotoxic T lymphocytes) are specific to the allelic peptides (Bucci *et al.* 2000). This suggests that these acquired allele-specific responses may be protective, and this may maintain the amino acid alleles in a frequency-dependent manner. Further work is needed to identify the nature of selection on LSA-1 sequences, as the results would be relevant to design of a *P. falciparum* vaccine containing LSA-1 (Kurtis *et al.* 2001).

In contrast, the McDonald-Kreitman analysis shows no evidence of selection on *csp* (the gene encoding the circumsporozoite protein), although the dN/dS ratio within *P. falciparum* alone has been taken as evidence for positive selection (Table 3). Which result should be accepted, or can they be reconciled? As with any single type of analysis, the McDonald-Kreitman test will be able to identify a real non-neutral pattern of sequence polymorphism in some cases, but not others. For example, it could be that there is positive diversifying selection on the *csp* gene causing adaptive changes between species as well as allelic differences within species, and both effects would cancel out the ability of the McDonald-Kreitman test to detect either. Immunological studies have clearly shown T cell responses to allele-specific peptide sequences of the CSP (Zevering, Khamboonruang & Good, 1994; Gilbert *et al.* 1998; Plebanski *et al.* 1999) and have led to the hypothesis that these maintain an adaptive polymorphism, either by escape or by antagonism (Gilbert *et al.* 1998; Plebanski *et al.* 1999). However, it is not known whether these particular responses are effective in killing parasites, and there is evidence that most protective responses to the CSP-based RTS,S/AS02 vaccine are not allele-specific (Bojang *et al.* 2001). In this case, and in general, there is a need to perform further analyses to detect the precise type of selection operating.

MORE THAN ONE METHOD IS REQUIRED

There is a real possibility that some signatures of diversifying selection on pathogen antigens are not caused by immune responses. If the results of one test are taken in isolation, and caution not applied to the processes of hypothesis generation and testing, misleading conclusions are likely. The McDonald-Kreitman test in Table 4 shows evidence of diversifying selection on the *pfs48/45* gene (encoding a major component of the malaria parasite gametocyte and gamete surface) in *P. falciparum*. It would be incorrect to conclude from this that selection maintains variation within *P. falciparum* populations. The *pfs48/45* sequences were derived from isolates of scattered origin, rather than being sampled from one local population, so the result could be due to geographically divergent selection fixing different alleles in different populations (Fig. 2). Detailed studies of the distribution of *pfs48/45* alleles throughout the world show that they are more geographically skewed than alleles at any other locus

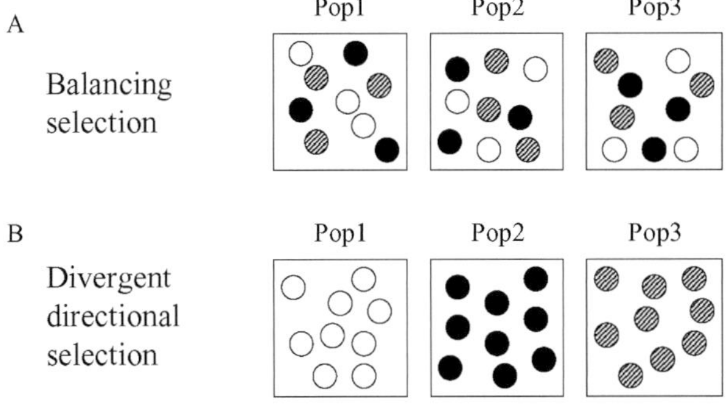

Fig. 2. Scheme of two cases of positive diversifying selection within a species, with completely opposite causes. A. Balancing selection maintains allelic diversity within populations (for example due to frequency-dependent selection favouring rare types). B. Divergent selection in different populations leads to fixation of different alleles (adaptation of populations to different conditions). Note that broad sampling of genotypes from the species would yield similar diversity in each case. Structured sampling of different populations would be required to reveal the distribution of the alleles and the likely cause of selection.

(Drakeley *et al.* 1996; Conway *et al.* 2001). This employs the F_{ST} index as listed in Table 3, with *pfs48/45* having exceptionally high values compared to other loci. This is the opposite to the result expected from balancing selection, and therefore does not lead to a hypothesis of allele specific immunity. A much more plausible hypothesis has emerged in this case, as the Pfs48/45 protein has a fertilisation role in the male gamete, and intense competition between male gametes is likely to drive adaptive changes (Conway *et al.* 2001; van Dijk *et al.* 2001).

Other antigen genes have yielded consistent evidence of balancing selection, maintaining variation within populations. The signatures of selection can be located in particular regions of the genes, and immune responses to the corresponding regions of the proteins can then be prospectively studied.

EVIDENCE OF IMMUNE SELECTION ON THE *P. FALCIPARUM* APICAL MEMBRANE ANTIGEN 1

The apical membrane antigen-1 gene (*ama1*) is present in a single copy in all *Plasmodium* species studied, and is also present in the distantly related apicomplexan *Toxoplasma gondii* (Hehl *et al.* 2000). There is sequence polymorphism in *ama1* of *P. falciparum*, which is markedly higher at non-synonymous compared to synonymous nucleotide sites (Hughes & Hughes, 1995; Verra & Hughes, 1999). The predominance of non-synonymous changes is particularly high among alleles of *P. falciparum*, when compared to inter-specific differences with *P. reichenowi* in the McDonald-Kreitman test, as noted in Table 4 (Kocken *et al.* 2000). This is highly significant for the surface-accessible 'ectodomain' region of the mature protein, but there is no effect seen in the region encoding the N-terminal 'signal and prosequence' which is cleaved prior to externalisation of the remainder of the protein on the merozoite surface (Kocken *et al.* 2000). Focusing on the sequence encoding the ectodomain, a large survey of alleles was then made from a single endemic population in Nigeria, and multiple tests were applied to locate any non-neutral effects more precisely. Figure 3 shows a sliding window plot along the sequence for indices of neutrality (Tajima's and Fu & Li's). Departure from neutrality was significant, with strongest evidence of diversifying selection (the most positive values of Tajima's and Fu & Li's indices) on domains I and III of the sequence (Polley & Conway, 2001).

It was thus predicted that acquired protective immune responses exist against allele-specific epitopes in the *P. falciparum* AMA1 protein, particularly in Domains I and III. Direct evidence of this has emerged from recent assays of parasite invasion inhibition by human antibodies affinity-purified to one allelic form of AMA1 (3D7 type), and by antibodies from a rabbit immunised with that allelic form (Hodder *et al.* 2001). Homologous (3D7) parasites were highly inhibited by both antibody preparations, but parasites with a divergent AMA1 allele sequence (HB3 type) were less effectively inhibited. Another heterologous parasite (D10) had a sequence more similar to 3D7 (being identical in Domain I), and this was very effectively inhibited, suggesting that inhibitory antibodies recognise allele-specific sequences in Domain I (Hodder, Crewther & Anders, 2001). Further work is required to investigate whether there are inhibitory antibodies to Domain III.

EVIDENCE OF IMMUNE SELECTION ON THE *P. FALCIPARUM* MEROZOITE SURFACE PROTEIN 1

The merozoite surface protein 1 (MSP1) is encoded by a single copy gene in all *Plasmodium* parasites, with a high level of sequence polymorphism in each species studied. In *P. falciparum*, more than 30% of the amino acid residues differ among naturally occurring alleles (Miller *et al.* 1993), although there are a few regions of the protein sequence in which less than 10% of residues are polymorphic (such as the c-terminal $MSP1_{19}$ fragment). Immunisation with purified MSP1 has conferred a significant level of protection to blood-stage challenge in New World Monkeys (Hall *et al.* 1984; Siddiqui *et al.* 1987), and it is considered essential to identify the targets of protective antibodies in this model and also in naturally acquired human immunity. Much attention has been focused on the c-terminal $MSP1_{19}$, which is a major target of antibodies that inhibit invasion *in vitro* (Patino *et al.* 1997; O'Donnell *et al.*

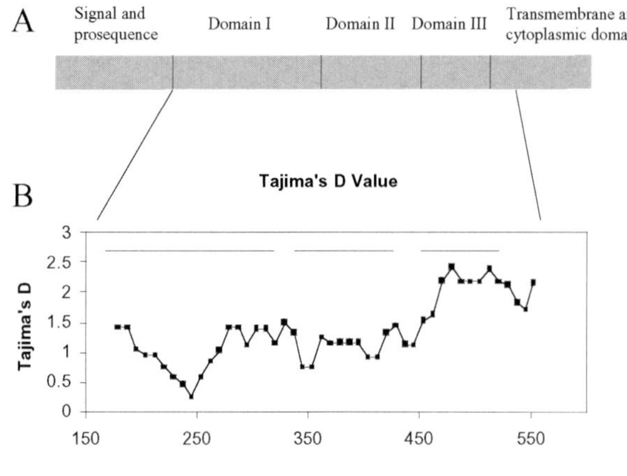

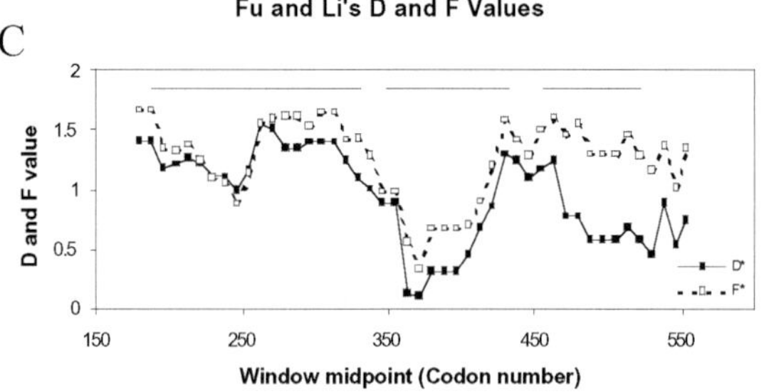

Fig. 3. Scheme of *Plasmodium falciparum ama1* with two sliding window tests of neutrality, using a sample of 51 alleles randomly taken from one population in Nigeria. A. Block scheme showing the major domains of the protein (Domain I–III together comprise the merozoite surface-accessible 'ectodomain' of the mature protein). B. Sliding window plots Tajima's D index (positive values indicate balancing selection, negative would indicate directional selection). C. Sliding window of Fu & Li's D and F indices (positive values indicate balancing selection, negative would indicate directional selection). Horizontal lines at the top of panels B and C show the positions of Domains I–III.

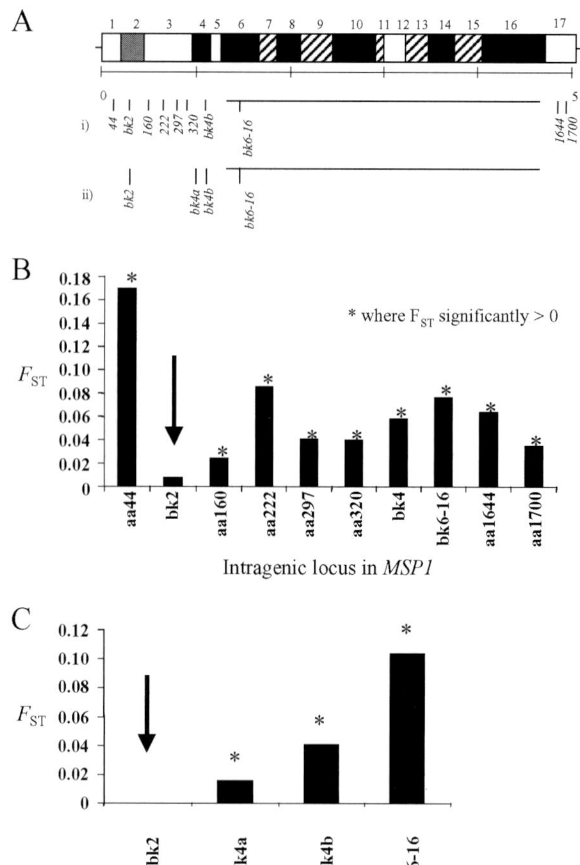

Fig. 4. A. Scheme of the *P. falciparum msp1* gene (blocks with solid shading have the most, diagonal shading intermediate, and no shading the least amino acid polymorphisms; Tanabe *et al.* 1987). Below are (i) 10 polymorphic sites studied in 6 population samples from Africa, (ii) 4 polymorphic sites studied in 2 populations in Southeast Asia (Conway *et al.* 2000*a*). B. Summary of F_{ST} indices (the proportion of overall allelic variation which differs among populations) for the 10 polymorphic sites (intragenic loci) among the 6 populations in Africa. C. Summary of F_{ST} indices for the 4 polymorphic sites among the 2 populations in Southeast Asia. Asterisks show where F_{ST} values were significantly > 0. Arrows indicate the particular site in the gene (*block 2*, abbreviated to *bk2*) with the lowest F_{ST} index in both continental analyses (i.e. at which most of the overall diversity is also represented within each local population).

2001). The remainder of the protein has been much less intensively studied.

Alleles of the *P. falciparum msp1* gene exist at stable frequencies over time in highly endemic populations (Conway, Greenwood & McBride, 1992; Ferreira *et al.* 1998), although they are less stable in epidemic or low-endemic populations (Babiker, Satti & Walliker, 1995; Silva *et al.* 2000). To investigate whether polymorphism in any single part of *msp1* is under particularly strong balancing selection, polymorphic sites in different parts of the gene (Fig. 4A) were typed in multiple population samples from endemic areas in Africa and Southeast Asia, and the allele frequency distributions analysed. Of the 10 polymorphic sites studied in the 6 African populations, the one with the lowest geographical variance (F_{ST}) in frequencies among populations (i.e. the polymorphic site at which most of the overall diversity exists also within each of the local populations) was *block 2* (*bk2*, Fig. 4B). Also, of the 4 polymorphic sites studied in the two Southeast Asian populations, *block 2* had the most similar allele frequencies in both populations and thus the lowest F_{ST} value (Fig. 4C).

From these results, it was predicted that allele-specific protective immune responses occur against the block 2 part of the MSP1 protein, causing balancing selection which maintains alleles within populations. To test this, a cohort of Gambian children was studied for serum antibody reactivities to different recombinant proteins representing different allelic forms of block 2. The antibody reactivities prior to the annual malaria transmission

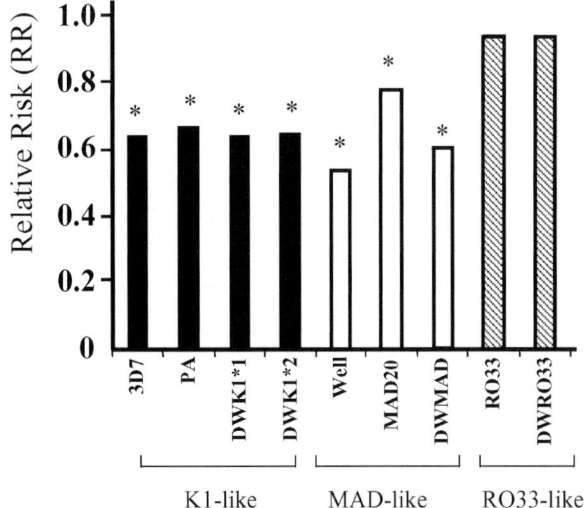

Fig. 5. Associations of anti-MSP1 block 2 antibodies with protection from clinical malaria in a longitudinal cohort study of Gambian children (data from Conway *et al.* 2000*a*). Reactivity of IgG in serum from 337 Gambian children in June (prior to the malaria transmission season) was tested for positivity by ELISA against a panel of 9 recombinant proteins representing block 2 sequences which fall into 3 major types (K1-like, MAD-like, and RO33-like; these have local allele frequencies in The Gambia of 0·51, 0·33 and 0·16, respectively). This positivity was tested for association with the subsequent experience of clinical malaria in these children from July–November (throughout the transmission season). A relative risk of < 1 indicates where antibody reactivity is associated with a reduced risk of malaria (asterisks show where this is statistically significant).

season were tested as predictors of an outcome of clinical malaria at any point during follow up throughout the malaria season. Antibodies against any of the recombinant proteins representing the two most frequent allelic types of block 2 in The Gambia (K1-like and MAD20-like) were strongly associated with a lower prospective risk of clinical malaria (relative risks of significantly < 1·0, Fig. 5). Children with antibodies against both K1-like and MAD20-like types had an even lower risk of malaria, consistent with the additive effect expected with allele-specific immunity (Conway *et al.* 2000*a*). Antibodies to the rarest of the block 2 types (RO33-like) were not significantly associated with protection.

PATHOGENS WITH EPIDEMIC POPULATIONS

The studies of *P. falciparum* that form the above examples have utilised the fact that this pathogen shows quite stable endemicity throughout much of its range, particularly in Africa. The acquisition of non-sterile protective immunity with repeated exposure throughout life is a characteristic feature of the epidemiology, as is the temporal stability of the frequency distributions of antigen types. These features are characteristic of many endemic pathogens apart from malaria parasites, including some of those causing diseases of human and veterinary importance. In contrast, there are many pathogens which inflict most clinical disease during epidemics. Those which cause only rare or sporadic human outbreaks, such as *Cryptosporidium parvum* (Fayer, Morgan & Upton, 2000) or Ebola virus (Oyok *et al.* 2001), are not maintained within the population and it is likely that human immune selection plays only a minor role in their evolution.

However, pathogens which cause regular human epidemics, and those which are normally maintained asymptomatically in humans (with 'emergence' of symptomatic cases at some times and places), are likely to be under immune selection. Indeed, distinct antigenic types evolve, for example in *Neisseria meningitidis* group A (Zhu *et al.* 2001) and *Streptococcus* group A (Hoe *et al.* 1999; Kaplan, Wotton & Johnson, 2001) and human immune selection can cause a replacement of a previous antigenic type with a new one rather than maintenance of a polymorphism. Such positive selection of new types causes alleles to go towards fixation leading to a different signature of selection at the DNA level compared with selection that favours rare types regardless of their age. In other words, important antigens of common epidemic pathogens are more likely to be under directional selection, and those of common endemic pathogens are more likely to be under balancing selection. For epidemic pathogens, the direction and magnitude of allele frequency changes over time are important parameters to measure, as well as the frequency distributions of alleles in different populations at one time. If the replacement of antigen types is measurable over contemporary or recent historical time, phylogenetic analyses of the evolution of the antigen genes may be structured in relation to known epidemiological or infection events (Zhu *et al.* 2001). In these cases, such analyses can yield more efficient information than gene frequency based analyses, as more information can potentially be derived from a given amount of sequence information (Zanotto *et al.* 1999; Nielsen, 2001).

PHYLOGENETIC CONSIDERATIONS

A general method for detecting selection in phylogenies involves a maximum likelihood approach, using codon-based models of nucleotide substitution (reviewed by Yang & Bielawski, 2000). This can account for different nucleotide transition/transversion ratios and codon bias when calculating the number of potential synonymous and nonsynonymous sites in the data set. The models operate at the level of instantaneous changes between codons which are identified from phylogenetic trees representing the various sequences in the data set. Thus the analytical models can allow for variable selection

Table 5. Pathogen genes studied by Phylogenetic Analysis using Maximum Likelihood (PAML) to look for evidence of positive selection

Gene	Positive selection	Estimates of ω parameters (dN/dS ratio classes) where positive selection shown
Dengue Virus *E-glycoprotein* gene	No	n/a
Human influenza virus A *hemagglutinin* (HA) gene	Yes	$\omega_0 = 0{\cdot}049$, $\omega_1 = 1{\cdot}284$, $\omega_2 = 6{\cdot}898$
HIV-1 *vif* gene	Yes	$\omega_0 = 0{\cdot}108$, $\omega_1 = 1{\cdot}211$, $\omega_2 = 4{\cdot}024$
HIV-1 *pol* gene	Yes	$\omega_0 = 0{\cdot}049$, $\omega_1 = 0{\cdot}849$, $\omega_2 = 4{\cdot}739$
HIV-1 *env* gene	Yes	$\omega_0 = 0{\cdot}175$, $\omega_1 = 1{\cdot}781$, $\omega_2 = 7{\cdot}141$
Japanese encephalitis *env* gene	No	n/a
Tick-borne flavivirus *NS5* gene	No	n/a

Analyses are from Yang *et al.* (2000). The selection model used allows codon sites to fall into three distinct classes with regards to dN/dS ratio. Where positive selection was evident the dN/dS (ω) value of each of the three site classes is shown. Where the dN/dS ratio of a class of sites is greater than 1, this indicates that there are codons under diversifying selection. n/a, not applicable (where models did not support positive selection).

intensities amongst codon sites, where not all sites in the sequence will have the same dN/dS ratio. This is important as many codons in a sequence are likely to be under negative or purifying selection (where mutations are deleterious and selected against) and thus have a dN/dS ratio of less than 1, and the method is therefore capable of detecting sites under positive selection even against this background of negative selection operating at other sites within the gene. In contrast, other methods which calculate dN/dS give an average ratio for all sites analysed and so are more greatly influenced by negative selection.

The maximum likelihood approach applies a series of models to the data set including models which incorporate selection, and assigns a likelihood value to each model allowing comparison between models. This maximum likelihood approach has been used to test for positive selection in several pathogen genes (Table 5). A problem arises where recombination is evident in a data set, as no single branching phylogeny will be accurate for all polymorphic sites (a net-like structure would best show the relationship between gene sequences). There is some indication that the method is not greatly affected by different possible alternative tree morphologies (Yang *et al.* 2000), but the use of any single phylogeny in these cases will cause some individual sites to be over-sampled, as they will appear on more than one branch due to recombination. Care must be taken therefore to assess the level of recombination in a data set before applying this or other phylogenetic analyses and interpreting their outcome.

Where high levels of recombination exist, making the formation of an accurate intra-specific phylogeny impossible, an *ad hoc* method which includes information on codon bias but not on phylogenetic structure may be attempted (Yang & Nielsen, 2000). This is less powerful than the phylogenetic approach, as it assigns an overall dN/dS value which is the average across all sites and will therefore be affected by a background of negative selection. However, this retains the discriminatory feature of rejecting dN/dS ratios of > 1 which are the result of codon bias rather than positive selection. For parasites such as *P. falciparum* (very high A/T content) and *Toxoplasma gondii* (very high G/C content) this may prove a useful approach.

It is relevant to note that many pathogens have probably become common in human populations quite recently, and contain only a very low overall level of nucleotide variation today. These include viral (Zanotto *et al.* 1996), bacterial (Sreevatsan *et al.* 1997; Achtman *et al.* 1999), and protozoan (Rich *et al.* 1998; Conway *et al.* 2000*b*; Volkman *et al.* 2001) examples. Some diseases caused by these pathogens have been known for hundreds or thousands of years, so they are not necessarily recent in an epidemiological or historic sense. However, an origin in the order of tens of thousands of years ago is still evolutionarily recent and can have an impact on current population structure and the choice of tests for selection, but is not likely to be a general disadvantage. Expanding populations tend to have an excess of rare new alleles and fewer at intermediate frequencies compared to older populations at mutation-drift equilibrium (Li, 1997). This will cause an opposite effect on nucleotide frequency distributions to that caused by balancing selection, so frequency-based tests such as Tajima's (Tajima, 1989) will be conservative (i.e. a positive inference of balancing selection is likely to be robust). Intra-specific phylogenies will be shallow, but otherwise will be as robust (or non-robust depending on the amount of recombination) as in older species. Moreover, a low background of nucleotide diversity means that broadly surveying genomes for regions of high diversity could be a useful screening procedure, allowing particular loci to be chosen for further work. The evaluation of extensive or intensive means of identifying pathogen loci under immune selection is an ongoing priority for infectious disease research.

REFERENCES

ACHTMAN, M., ZURTH, K., MORELLI, G., TORREA, G., GUIYOULE, A. & CARNIEL, E. (1999). *Yersinia pestis*, the cause of plague, is a recently emerged clone of *Yersinia pseudotuberculosis*. *Proceedings of The National Academy of Sciences, USA* **96**, 14043–14048.

AIDOO, M., LALVANI, A., ALLSOPP, C. E. M., PLEBANSKI, M., MEISNER, S. J., KRAUSA, P., BROWNING, M., MORRIS JONES, S., GOTCH, F., FIDOCK, D. A., TAKIGUCHI, M., ROBSON, K. J. H., GREENWOOD, B. M., DRUILHE, P., WHITTLE, H. C. & HILL, A. V. S. (1995). Identification of conserved antigenic components for a cytotoxic T lymphocyte-inducing vaccine against malaria. *Lancet* **345**, 1003–1007.

ALLEN, T. M., O'CONNOR, D. H., JING, P., DZURIS, J. L., MOTHE, B. R., VOGEL, T. U., DUNPHY, E. & LLEBL, M. E. *et al.* (2000). Tat-specific cytotoxic T lymphocytes select for SIV escape variants during resolution of primary viraemia. *Nature* **407**, 386–390.

ALLRED, D. R., CARLTON, J. M. R., SATCHER, R. L., LONG, J. A., BROWN, W. C., PATTERSON, P. E., O'CONNOR, R. M. & STROUP, S. E. (2000). The *ves* multigene family of *B. bovis* encodes components of rapid antigenic variation at the infected erythrocyte surface. *Molecular Cell* **5**, 153–162.

ANDERSON, T. J. C. & DAY, K. P. (2000). Geographical structure and sequence evolution as inferred from the *Plasmodium falciparum S-antigen* locus. *Molecular and Biochemical Parasitology* **106**, 321–326.

BABIKER, H. A., SATTI, G. & WALLIKER, D. (1995). Genetic changes in the population of *Plasmodium falciparum* in a Sudanese village over a three year period. *American Journal of Tropical Medicine and Hygiene* **53**, 7–15.

BINKS, R. H., BAUM, J., ODUOLA, A. M. J., ARNOT, D. E., BABIKER, H. A., KREMSNER, P. G., ROPER, C., GREENWOOD, B. M. & CONWAY, D. J. (2001). Population genetic analysis of the *Plasmodium falciparum* erythrocyte binding antigen-175 (*eba-175*) gene. *Molecular and Biochemical Parasitology* **114**, 63–70.

BOJANG, K. A., MILLIGAN, P. J. M., PINDER, M., VIGNERON, L., ALLOUECHE, A., KESTER, K. E., BALLOU, W. R., CONWAY, D. J., REECE, W. H. H., GOTHARD, P., YAMUAH, L., DELCHAMBRE, M., VOSS, G., GREENWOOD, B. M., HILL, A., MCADAM, K. P. W. J., TORNIEPORTH, N., COHEN, J. D. & DOHERTY, T. (2001). Efficacy of RTS,S/AS02 malaria vaccine against *Plasmodium falciparum* infection in semi-immune adult men in The Gambia: a randomised trial. *Lancet* **358**, 1927–1934.

BORST, P. & ULBERT, S. (2001). Control of VSG expression sites. *Molecular and Biochemical Parasitology* **114**, 17–27.

BRAYTON, K. A., KNOWLES, D. P., MCGUIRE, T. C. & PALMER, G. H. (2001). Efficient use of a small genome to generate antigenic diversity in tick-borne ehrlichial pathogens. *Proceedings of the National Academy of Sciences, USA* **98**, 4130–4135.

BUCCI, K., KASTENS, W., HOLLINGDALE, M. R., SHANKAR, A., ALPERS, M. P., KING, C. L. & KAZURA, J. W. (2000). Influence of age and HLA type on interferon-gamma (IFN-gamma) responses to a naturally occurring polymorphic epitope of *Plasmodium falciparum* liver stage antigen-1 (LSA-1). *Clinical and Experimental Immunology* **122**, 94–100.

CONWAY, D. J. (1997). Natural selection on polymorphic malaria antigens and the search for a vaccine. *Parasitology Today* **13**, 26–29.

CONWAY, D. J., CAVANAGH, D. R., TANABE, K., ROPER, C., MIKES, Z. S., SAKIHAMA, N., BOJANG, K. A., ODUOLA, A. M. J., KREMSNER, P. G., ARNOT, D. E., GREENWOOD, B. M. & MCBRIDE, J. S. (2000*a*). A principal target of human immunity to malaria identified by molecular population genetic and immunological analyses. *Nature Medicine* **6**, 689–692.

CONWAY, D. J., FANELLO, C., LLOYD, J. M., AL-JOUBORI, B. M. A.-S., BALOCH, A. H., SOMANATH, S. D., ROPER, C., ODUOLA, A. M. J., MULDER, B., POVOA, M. M., SINGH, B. & THOMAS, A. W. (2000*b*). Origin of *Plasmodium falciparum* malaria is traced by mitochondrial DNA. *Molecular and Biochemical Parasitology* **111**, 163–171.

CONWAY, D. J., GREENWOOD, B. M. & MCBRIDE, J. S. (1992). Longitudinal study of *Plasmodium falciparum* polymorphic antigens in a malaria endemic population. *Infection and Immunity* **60**, 1122–1127.

CONWAY, D. J., MACHADO, R. L. D., SINGH, B., DESSERT, P., MIKES, Z. S., POVOA, M. M., ODUOLA, A. M. J. & ROPER, C. (2001). Extreme geographical fixation of variation in the *Plasmodium falciparum* gamete surface protein gene Pfs48/45 compared with microsatellite loci. *Molecular and Biochemical Parasitology* **115**, 145–156.

DRAKELEY, C. J., DURAISINGH, M. T., POVOA, M., CONWAY, D. J., TARGETT, G. A. T. & BAKER, D. A. (1996). Geographical distribution of a variant epitope of Pfs48/45, a *Plasmodium falciparum* transmission-blocking vaccine candidate. *Molecular and Biochemical Parasitology* **81**, 253–257.

ESCALANTE, A. A., LAL, A. A. & AYALA, F. J. (1998). Genetic polymorphism and natural selection in the malaria parasite *Plasmodium falciparum*. *Genetics* **149**, 189–202.

EVANS, D. T., O'CONNOR, D. H., JING, P., DZURIS, J. L., SIDNEY, J., DA SILVA, J., ALLEN, T. M., HORTON, H., VENHAM, J. E., RUDERSDORF, R. A., VOGEL, T., PAUZA, C. D., BONTROP, R. E., DEMARS, R., SETTE, A., HUGHES, A. L. & WATKINS, D. I. (1999). Virus-specific cytotoxic T lymphocyte responses select for amino-acid variation in simian immunodeficiency virus Env and Nef. *Nature Medicine* **5**, 1270–1276.

FAYER, R., MORGAN, U. & UPTON, S. J. (2000). Epidemiology of *Cryptosporidium*: transmission, detection, and identification. *International Journal for Parasitology* **30**, 1305–1322.

FELGER, I., MARSHALL, V. M., REEDER, J. C., HUNT, J. A., MGONE, C. S. & BECK, H.-P. (1997). Sequence diversity and molecular evolution of the merozoite surface antigen 2 of *Plasmodium falciparum*. *Journal of Molecular Evolution* **45**, 154–160.

FERREIRA, M. U., LIU, Q., ZHOU, M., KIMURA, M., KANEKO, O., VAN THIEN, H., ISOMURA, S., TANABE, K. & KAWAMOTO, F. (1998). Stable patterns of allelic diversity at the merozoite surface protein-1 locus of *Plasmodium falciparum* in clinical isolates from southern Vietnam. *Journal of Eukaryotic Microbiology* **45**, 131–136.

FIDOCK, D. A., GRAS-MASSE, H., LEPERS, J. P., BRAHIMI, K., BENMOHAMED, L., MELLOUK, S., GUERIN-MARCHAND, C., LONDONO, A., RAHARIMALALA, L., MEIS, J. F., LANGSLEY, G., ROUSSILHON, C., TARTAR, A. & DRUILHE, P. (1994). *Plasmodium falciparum* liver stage antigen-1 is well conserved and contains potent B and T cell determinants. *Journal of Immunology* **153**, 190–204.

FU, Y.-X. & LI, W.-H. (1993). Statistical tests of neutrality of mutations. *Genetics* **133**, 693–709.

FUDYK, T. C., MACLEAN, I. W., SIMONSEN, J. N., NJAGI, E. N., KIMANI, J., BRUNHAM, R. C. & PLUMMER, F. A. (1999). Genetic diversity and mosaicism at the *por* locus of *Neisseria gonorrhoeae*. *Journal of Bacteriology* **181**, 5591–5599.

GILBERT, S. C., PLEBANSKI, M., GUPTA, S., MORRIS, J., COX, M., AIDOO, M., KWIATKOWSKI, D., GREENWOOD, B. M., WHITTLE, H. C. & HILL, A. V. S. (1998). Association of malaria parasite population structure, HLA, and immunological antagonism. *Science* **279**, 1173–1177.

GOULDER, P. J. R., BRANDER, C., TANG, Y., TREMBLAY, C., COLBERT, R. A., ADDO, M. M., ROSENBERG, E. S., NGUYEN, T., ALLEN, R., TROCHA, A., ALTFELD, M., HE, S. Q., BUNCE, M., FUNKHOUSER, R., PELTON, S. I., BURCHETT, S. K., MCINTOSH, K., KORBER, B. T. M. & WALKER, B. D. (2001). Evolution and transmission of stable CTL escape mutations in HIV infection. *Nature* **412**, 334–338.

GUBBELS, M.-J, KATZER, F., HIDE, G., JONGEJAN, F. & SHIELS, B. R. (2000). Generation of a mosaic pattern of diversity in the major merozoite-piroplasm surface antigen of *Theileria annulata*. *Molecular and Biochemical Parasitology* **110**, 23–32.

HALL, R., HYDE, J. E., GOMAN, M., SIMMONS, D. L., HOPE, I. A., MACKAY, M., SCAIFE, J., MERKLI, B., RICHLE, R. & STOCKER, J. (1984). Major surface antigen gene of a human malaria parasite cloned and expressed in bacteria. *Nature* **311**, 379–382.

HAY, C. M., RUHL, D. J., BASGOZ, N. O., WILSON, C. C., BILLINGSLEY, J. M., DEPASQUALE, M. P., D'AQUILA, R. T., WOLINSKY, S. M., CRAWFORD, J. M., MONTEFIORI, D. C. & WALKER, B. D. (1999). Lack of viral escape and defective *in vivo* activation of human immunodeficiency virus type 1-specific cytotoxic T lymphocytes in rapidly progressive infection. *Journal of Virology* **73**, 5509–5519.

HEHL, A. B., LEKUTIS, C., GRIGG, M. E., BRADLEY, P. J., DUBREMETZ, J.-F., ORTEGA-BARRIA, E. & BOOTHROYD, J. C. (2000). *Toxoplasma gondii* homologue of *Plasmodium* apical membrane antigen 1 is involved in invasion of host cells. *Infection and Immunity* **68**, 7078–7076.

HODDER, A. N., CREWTHER, P. E. & ANDERS, R. F. (2001). Specificity of the protective antibody response to apical membrane antigen 1. *Infection and Immunity* **69**, 3286–3294.

HOE, N. P., NAKASHIMA, K., LUKOMSKI, S., GRIGSBY, D., LIU, M., KORDARI, P. & DOU, S.-J. *et al.* (1999). Rapid selection of complement-inhibiting protein variants in group A *Streptococcus* epidemic waves. *Nature Medicine* **5**, 924–929.

HOFFMAN, E. H. E., DA SILVEIRA, L. A., TONHOSOLO, R., PEREIRA, F. J. T., RIBEIRO, W. L., TONON, A. P., KAWAMOTO, F. & FERREIRA, M. U. (2001). Geographical patterns of allelic diversity in the *Plasmodium falciparum* malaria vaccine candidate, merozoite surface protein-2. *Annals of Tropical Medicine and Parasitology* **95**, 117–132.

HUGHES, M. K. & HUGHES, A. L. (1995). Natural selection on *Plasmodium* surface proteins. *Molecular and Biochemical Parasitology* **71**, 99–113.

KAPLAN, E. L., WOTTON, J. T. & JOHNSON, D. R. (2001). Dynamic epidemiology of group A streptococcal serotypes associated with pharyngitis. *Lancet* **358**, 1334–1337.

KELLEHER, A. D., LONG, C., HOLMES, E. C., ALLEN, R. L., WILSON, J., CONLON, C., WORKMAN, C., SHAUNAK, S., OLSON, K., GOULDER, P., BRANDER, C., OGG, G., SULLIVAN, J. S., DYER, W., JONES, I., MCMICHAEL, A. J., ROWLAND-JONES, S. & PHILLIPS, R. E. (2001). Clustered mutations in HIV-1 gag are consistently required for escape from HLA-B27-restricted cytotoxic T lymphocyte responses. *Journal of Experimental Medicine* **193**, 375–385.

KIMURA, M. (1983). *The Neutral Theory of Molecular Evolution*. Cambridge, Cambridge University Press.

KOCKEN, C. H. M., NARUM, D. L., MASSOUGBODJI, A., AYIVI, B., DUBBELD, M. A., VAN DER WEL, A., CONWAY, D. J., SANNI, A. & THOMAS, A. W. (2000). Molecular characterisation of *Plasmodium reichenowi* apical membrane antigen-1 (AMA-1), comparison with *P. falciparum* AMA-1, and antibody-mediated inhibition of red cell invasion. *Molecular and Biochemical Parasitology* **109**, 147–156.

KREITMAN, M. (2000). Methods to detect selection in populations with application to the human. *Annual Review of Genomics and Human Genetics* **1**, 539–559.

KURTIS, J. D., HOLLINGDALE, M. R., LUTY, A. J. F., LANAR, D. E., KRZYCH, U. & DUFFY, P. E. (2001). Pre-erythrocytic immunity to *Plasmodium falciparum*: the case for an LSA-1 vaccine. *Trends in Parasitology* **17**, 219–223.

LI, W.-H. (1997). *Molecular Evolution*. Sunderland, Mass, Sinauer Associates, Inc.

MARTIENSSEN, R. A. & COLOT, V. (2001). DNA methylation and epigenetic inheritance in plants and filamentous fungi. *Science* **293**, 1070–1074.

MCCOLL, D. J. & ANDERS, R. F. (1997). Conservation of structural motifs and antigenic diversity in *Plasmodium falciparum* merozoite surface protein-3 (MSP-3). *Molecular and Biochemical Parasitology* **90**, 21–31.

MCDONALD, J. H. (1994). Detecting natural selection by comparing geographic variation in protein and DNA polymorphisms. In *Non-Neutral Evolution: Theories and Molecular Data* (ed. Golding, B.), pp. 88–100. Chapman & Hall, New York & London.

MCDONALD, J. H. & KREITMAN, M. (1991). Adaptive protein evolution at the *Adh* locus in *Drosophila*. *Nature* **351**, 652–654.

MEHR, I. J., LONG, C. D., SERKIN, C. D. & SEIFERT, H. S. (2000). A homologue of the recombination-dependent growth gene, *rdgC*, is involved in gonococcal pilin antigenic variation. *Genetics* **154**, 523–532.

MILLER, L. H., ROBERTS, T., SHAHABUDDIN, M. & MCCUTCHAN, T. F. (1993). Analysis of sequence diversity in the *Plasmodium falciparum* merozoite surface protein-1 (MSP-1). *Molecular and Biochemical Parasitology* **59**, 1–14.

NEI, M. & GOJOBORI, T. (1986). Simple methods for estimating the numbers of synonymous and nonsynonymous substitutions. *Molecular Biology and Evolution* **3**, 418–426.

NIELSEN, R. (2001). Statistical tests of selective neutrality in the age of genomics. *Heredity* **86**, 641–647.

O'DONNELL, R., DE KONING-WARD, T. F., BURT, R. A., BOCKAIRE, M., REEDER, J. C., COWMAN, A. F. & CRABB, B. S. (2001). Antibodies against merozoite surface protein (MSP)-1 19 are a major component of the invasion-inhibitory response in individuals immune to malaria. *Journal of Experimental Medicine* **193**, 1403–1412.

OKENU, D. M. N., THOMAS, A. W. & CONWAY, D. J. (2000). Allelic lineages of the merozoite surface protein 3 (msp3) gene in *Plasmodium reichenowi* and *Plasmodium falciparum*. *Molecular and Biochemical Parasitology* **109**, 185–188.

OYOK, T., ODONGA, C., MULWANI, E., ABUR, J., KADUCU, F., AKECH, M., OLANGO, J. & ONEK, P. *et al.* (2001). Outbreak of Ebola Hemorrhagic Fever – Uganda, August 2000–January 2001. *Journal of the American Medical Association* **285**, 1010–1012.

OZWARA, H., KOCKEN, C. H. M., CONWAY, D. J., MWENDA, J. M. & THOMAS, A. W. (2001). Comparative analysis of *Plasmodium reichenowi* and *P. falciparum* erythrocyte-binding proteins reveals selection to maintain polymorphism in the erythrocyte-binding region of EBA-175. *Molecular and Biochemical Parasitology* **116**, 81–84.

PARKHILL, J., WREN, B. W., MUNGALL, K., KETLEY, J. M., CHURCHER, C., BASHAM, D., CHILLINGWORTH, T., DAVIES, R. M., FELTWELL, T., HOLROYD, S., JAGELS, K., KARLYSHEV, A. V., MOULE, S., PALLEN, M. J., PENN, C. W., QUAIL, M. A., RAJANDREAM, M. A., RUTHERFORD, K. M., VAN VLIET, A. H. M., WHITEHEAD, S. & BARRELL, B. G. (2000). The genome sequence of the food borne pathogen *Campylobacter jejuni* reveals hypervariable sequences. *Nature* **403**, 665–668.

PATINO, J. A., HOLDER, A. A., MCBRIDE, J. S. & BLACKMAN, M. J. (1997). Antibodies that inhibit malaria merozoite surface protein-1 processing and erythrocyte invasion are blocked by naturally acquired human antibodies. *Journal of Experimental Medicine* **186**, 1689–1699.

PLEBANSKI, M., LEE, E. A. M., HANNAN, C. M., FLANAGAN, K. L., GILBERT, S. C., GRAVENOR, M. B. & HILL, A. V. S. (1999). Altered peptide ligands narrow the repertoire of cellular immune responses by interfering with T-cell priming. *Nature Medicine* **5**, 565–571.

POLLEY, S. D. & CONWAY, D. J. (2001). Strong diversifying selection on domains of the *Plasmodium falciparum* Apical Membrane Antigen 1 gene. *Genetics* **158**, 1505–1512.

PREISER, P. R., JARRA, W., CAPIOD, T. & SNOUNOU, G. (1999). A rhoptry-protein-associated mechanism of clonal phenotypic variation in rodent malaria. *Nature* **398**, 618–622.

RANNALA, B., QIU, W. G. & DYKHUIZEN, D. E. (2000). Methods for estimating gene frequencies and detecting selection in bacterial populations. *Genetics* **155**, 499–508.

RICH, S. M., LICHT, M. C., HUDSON, R. R. & AYALA, F. J. (1998). Malaria's eve: Evidence of a recent population bottleneck throughout the world populations of *Plasmodium falciparum*. *Proceedings of the National Academy of Sciences, USA* **95**, 4425–4430.

SIDDIQUI, W. A., TAM, L. Q., KRAMER, K. J., HUI, G. S. N., CASE, S. E., YAMAGA, K. M., CHANG, S. P., CHAN, E. B. T. & KAN, S.-C. (1987). Merozoite surface coat precursor protein completely protects *Aotus* monkeys against *Plasmodium falciparum* malaria. *Proceedings of the National Academy of Sciences, USA* **84**, 3014–3018.

SILVA, N. S., SILVEIRA, L. A., MACHADO, R. L. D., POVOA, M. M. & FERREIRA, M. U. (2000). Temporal and spatial distribution of the variants of merozoite surface protein-1 (MSP-1) in *Plasmodium falciparum* populations in Brazil. *Annals of Tropical Medicine and Parasitology* **94**, 675–688.

SMITH, J. D., GAMAIN, B., BARUCH, D. I. & KYES, S. (2001). Decoding the language of *var* genes and *Plasmodium falciparum* sequestration. *Trends in Parasitology* **17**, 538–545.

SREEVATSAN, S., PAN, X., STOCKBAUER, K. E., CONNELL, N. D., KREISWIRTH, B. N., WHITTAM, T. S. & MUSSER, J. M. (1997). Restricted structural gene polymorphism in the *Mycobacterium tuberculosis* complex indicates evolutionarily recent global dissemination. *Proceedings of the National Academy of Sciences, USA* **94**, 9869–9874.

STEPHENS, R. S. & LAMMEL, C. J. (2001). *Chlamydia* outer membrane protein discovery using genomics. *Current Opinion in Microbiology* **4**, 16–20.

STOTHARD, D. R., BOGUSLAWSKI, G. & JONES, R. B. (1998). Phylogenetic analysis of the *Chlamydia trachomatis* major outer membrane protein and examination of potential pathogenic determinants. *Infection and Immunity* **66**, 3618–3625.

STRINGER, J. R. & KEELY, S. P. (2001). Genetics of surface antigen expression in *Pneumocystis carinii*. *Infection and Immunity* **69**, 627–639.

SUAREZ, C. E., FLORIN-CHRISTENSEN, M., HINES, S. A., PALMER, G. H., BROWN, W. C. & MCELWAIN, T. F. (2000). Characterization of allelic variation in the *Babesia bovis* merozoite surface antigen 1 (*MSA-1*) locus and identification of a cross-reactive inhibition-sensitive MSA-1 epitope. *Infection and Immunity* **68**, 6865–6870.

TAJIMA, F. (1989). Statistical method for testing the neutral mutation hypothesis by DNA polymorphism. *Genetics* **123**, 585–595.

TANABE, K., MACKAY, M., GOMAN, M. & SCAIFE, J. G. (1987). Allelic dimorphism in a surface antigen gene of the malaria parasite *Plasmodium falciparum*. *Journal of Molecular Biology* **195**, 273–287.

THEISEN, M., THOMAS, A. W. & JEPSEN, S. (2001). Cloning, nucleotide sequencing and analysis of the gene encoding the glutamate-rich protein (GLURP) from

Plasmodium falciparum. Molecular and Biochemical Parasitology **115**, 269–273.

TSUCHIYA, E., SUGAWARA, K., HONGO, S., MATSUZAKI, Y., MURAKI, Y., LI, Z. N. & NAKAMURA, K. (2001). Antigenic structure of the haemagglutinin of human influenza A/H2N2 virus. *Journal of General Virology* **82**, 2475–2484.

VAN DIJK, M. R., JANSE, C. J., THOMPSON, J., WATERS, A. P., BRAKS, J. A. M., DODEMONT, H. J., STUNNENBERG, H. G., VAN GEMERT, G.-J., SAUERWEIN, R. W. & ELING, W. (2001). A central role for P48/45 in malaria parasite male gamete fertility. *Cell* **104**, 153–164.

VERRA, F. & HUGHES, A. L. (1999). Evidence for ancient balanced polymorphism at the apical membrane antigen-1 (*AMA-1*) locus of *Plasmodium falciparum. Molecular and Biochemical Parasitology* **105**, 149–153.

VIDAL, N., PEETERS, V. N., MULANGA-KABEYA, C., NZILAMBI, N., ROBERTSON, D., ILUNGA, W., SEMA, H., TSHIMANGA, K., BONGO, B. & DELAPORTE, E. (2000). Unprecedented degree of human immunodeficiency virus type 1 (HIV-1) group M genetic diversity in the Democratic Republic of Congo suggests that the HIV-1 pandemic originated in Central Africa. *Journal of Virology* **74**, 10498–10507.

VISESHAKUL, N., KAMPER, S., BOWIE, M. V. & BARBET, A. F. (2000). Sequence and expression analysis of a surface antigen gene family of the rickettsia *Anaplasma marginale. Gene* **253**, 45–53.

VOLKMAN, S. K., BARRY, A. E., LYONS, E. J., NIELSEN, K. M., THOMAS, S. M., CHOI, M., THAKORE, S. S., DAY, K. P., WIRTH, D. F. & HARTL, D. L. (2001). Recent origin of *Plasmodium falciparum* from a single progenitor. *Science* **293**, 482–484.

WATTERSON, G. A. (1978). The homozygosity test of neutrality. *Genetics* **88**, 405–417.

YANG, Z. & BIELAWSKI, J. P. (2000). Statistical methods for detecting molecular adaptation. *Trends in Ecology and Evolution* **15**, 496–503.

YANG, Z. & NIELSEN, R. (2000). Estimating synonymous and nonsynonymous substitution rates under realistic evolutionary models. *Molecular Biology and Evolution* **17**, 32–43.

YANG, Z., NIELSEN, R., GOLDMAN, N. & PEDERSEN, A.-M. K. (2000). Codon-substitution models for heterogeneous selection pressure at amino acid sites. *Genetics* **155**, 431–449.

ZANOTTO, P. M. D., GOULD, E. A., GAO, G. F., HARVEY, P. H. & HOLMES, E. C. (1996). Population dynamics of flaviviruses revealed by molecular phylogenies. *Proceedings of the National Academy of Sciences, USA* **93**, 548–553.

ZANOTTO, P. M. D., KALLAS, E. G., DE SOUZA, R. F. & HOLMES, E. C. (1999). Genealogical evidence for positive selection in the *nef* gene of HIV-1. *Genetics* **153**, 1077–1089.

ZEVERING, Y., KHAMBOONRUANG, C. & GOOD, M. F. (1994). Natural amino acid polymorphisms of the circumsporozoite protein of *Plasmodium falciparum* abrogate specific human CD4+ T cell responsiveness. *European Journal of Immunology* **24**, 1418–1425.

ZHANG, J.-R. & NORRIS, S. J. (1998). Kinetics and *in vivo* induction of genetic variation of *vlsE* in *Borrelia burgdorferi. Infection and Immunity* **66**, 3689–3697.

ZHU, P., VAN DER ENDE, A., FALUSH, D., BRIESKE, N., MORELLI, G., LINZ, B., POPOVIC, T., SCHUURMAN, I. G. A., ADEGBOLA, R. A., ZURTH, K., GAGNEUX, S., PLATONOV, A. E., RIOU, J. Y., CAUGANT, D. A., NICOLAS, P. & ACHTMAN, M. (2001). Fit genotypes and escape variants of subgroup III *Neisseria meningitidis* during three pandemics of epidemic meningitis. *Proceedings of the National Academy of Sciences, USA* **98**, 5234–5239.

A perspective on clonal phenotypic (antigenic) variation in protozoan parasites

C. M. R. TURNER

Division of Infection and Immunity, Institute of Biomedical and Life Sciences, Joseph Black Building, University of Glasgow, Glasgow, G12 8QQ

SUMMARY

Intra-clonal phenotypic (antigenic) variation is used by many pathogens to evade the consequences of immune-mediated killing by mammalian hosts. In this substantially theoretical article, I emphasise that antigenic variation (*sensu stricto*) involves no change in genotype; its importance as a mechanism for promoting pathogen transmission and its polyphyletic origin. From a functional perspective, antigenic variation is constrained by the requirement to meet five conditions. These are: capability to express several antigens against which functional immunity predominates; capability to interact with the environment; mutually exclusive expression of variable antigens in each cell within an infection; mutually exclusive expression in the within-host pathogen population and the capability for population growth within a host. Meeting these conditions leads to chronicity of infection and high rates of hierarchical and reversible switching of expression between variable antigens. The organisation of hierarchical expression is discussed in some detail.

Key words: Antigenic variation; parasite evolution; pathogen evolution; *Plasmodium*; malaria; trypanosome.

INTRODUCTION

Several species of microorganisms undergo a form of intra-clonal phenotypic variation. Amongst these are some of the world's most important pathogens, notably those causing malaria and sleeping sickness. The molecules that vary in these pathogens are antigens crucially involved in recognition and clearance (or lack of it) by host immune responses and hence intra-clonal phenotypic variation is termed antigenic variation. Antigenic variation has deserved the considerable attention devoted to it for the last century, particularly by protozoologists. In the last 20 years however, marked features of the research effort on antigenic variation have been, to my mind, the focus on molecular mechanisms and the independence of the literature on different organisms. The focus on molecular machinery of these processes has been a reflection of the wider-scale revolution in molecular biology, was sorely needed and has been extremely successful. Success breeds success. Perhaps the best example of this is the literature on *Trypanosoma brucei* (for recent reviews see Borst *et al.* 1998; Cross, Wirtz & Navarro, 1998; Pays & Nolan, 1998; Barry & McCullough, 2001). The independence of the literature on different pathogens is partly a necessity and partly a reflection of the fact that cross-pathogen comparisons of molecular mechanisms of antigenic variation have not engendered notable progress (but for a thoughtful counter-example see Alred, 1998). The aim of this article is to redress the balance a little. By taking a holistic view of antigenic variation, I attempt to show that there are issues which could be productively addressed from an evolutionary perspective and where comparisons between organisms might be illuminating.

It is helpful at the outset to make a clear distinction between two senses of the term 'antigenic variation' when applied to pathogens. Antigenic variation, *sensu lato*, includes the classical genetic mechanisms of mutation and recombination for generating diversity. These mechanisms may have important consequences for effective immunity against parasites but they are much less so than the consequences of antigenic variation, *sensu stricto* which has, I would contend, evolved with the specific purpose of immune evasion. 'Purpose' in this context is taken to mean conferment of ecological advantage that is selectable by evolution. The distinction between the two senses is that the second involves no change in genotype. That is, the enzymatic and transcriptional machinery that enacts switching between variant antigens is heritable between generations as are genes encoding variant antigens. But, changes in expression of variant antigens are readily reversible within a cloned cell line and are *not* heritable. This article concerns antigenic variation *sensu stricto*.

ANTIGENIC VARIATION AND TRANSMISSION

The ecological advantage of antigenic variation to any parasite that evolves this system is almost certainly to promote transmission between hosts. There is remarkably little direct experimental evidence

Tel: 0141 330 6629. Fax: 0141 330 2041.
E-mail: m.turner@bio.gla.ac.uk

Parasitology (2002), **125**, S17–S23.
DOI: 10.1017/S0031182002002470 Printed in the United Kingdom

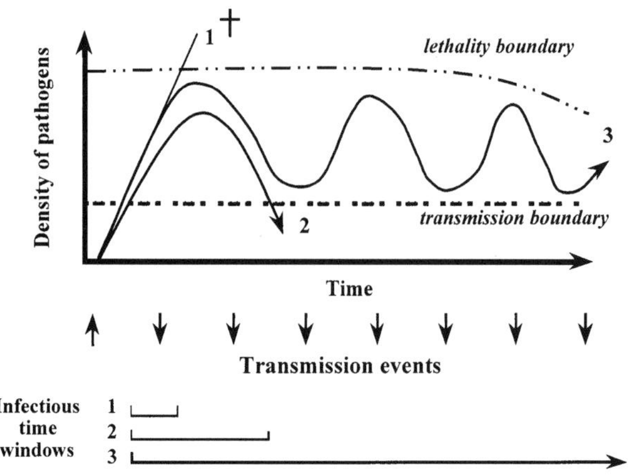

Fig. 1. A simplified diagrammatic representation of the relationship between antigenic variation and pathogen transmission. For explanation see text. Redrawn from Turner (1999).

linking antigenic variation with increased transmission but no serious alternative hypotheses to explain the evolution of antigenic variation have been put forward. Indirect evidence supporting the link between antigenic variation and transmission is of variable quality in different model systems but, in trypanosomes at least, the evidence is compelling (Turner, 1999). The link between antigenic variation and transmission is illustrated in Fig. 1. The key features in this highly simplified view of an infection are determined by the relationship of the course of infection to two boundaries – an upper 'lethality boundary' and a lower 'transmission boundary' and assume that transmission is dependent on pathogen density within an infected host. There is potential for successful transmission to another host only when the density is between the two boundaries. In scenario 1 in Fig. 1, there is no control of pathogen growth, the lethality boundary is breached leading to death of the host and curtailing transmission to a very short time window. In scenario 2, an immune response resolves the infection and there is an increase in the transmission window. Antigenic variation occurs in scenario 3 and maintains the pathogen density between the two boundaries for a longer time period thus causing a consequently greater increase in the transmission window.

Antigenic variation succeeds in extending an infection because there is a time delay between expression of an antigen and the development of a functional immune response against it. A 'functional' response would be one with cytotoxic or cytostatic effect on the pathogen, as opposed to a bystander response for example. During this time delay there is the opportunity for switching from expression of one variable antigen to that of another. Thus, during the first wave of an infection the pathogen population might comprise mainly of cells expressing one type of variable antigen but with antigenic switching

Table 1. Protozoa in which clonal phenotypic (antigenic) variation *sensu stricto* has been suggested. This is not an exhaustive list, but does illustrate the diversity of genera and species that appear to use this process. The last two species listed are free-living, whereas the others are all parasites. The quality of evidence varies considerably between organisms. *indicates review

Species	Reference
Trypanosoma brucei	Barry & McCullough (2001)*
T. congolense	Masake *et al.* (1983)
T. vivax	Barry (1986)
T. evansi	Jones & McKinnell (1985)
Plasmodium falciparum	Craig & Scherf (2001)*
P. vivax	Del Portillo *et al.* (2001)
P. chabaudi	Phillips *et al.* (1997)*
P. fragile	Hadunetti *et al.* (1987)
P. knowlesi	Al-Khedery *et al.* (1999)
Babesia bovis	Alred *et al.* (2000)
Giardia lamblia	Svärd *et al.* (1998)
Paramecium aurelia complex	Caron & Meyer (1989)*
Tetrahymena thermophila	Preer (1986)*

occurring to generate a small sub-population expressing a different type. The immune response is directed against the numerically dominant type thus causing resolution of the first wave of infection, but this response is variable antigen-specific and thus ineffective against cells expressing other variable antigens which will grow causing recrudescence of infection as shown (Fig. 1, scenario 3). This process is repeated continually, dependent on the interaction between antigenic variation and population growth on the part of the pathogen and variable antigen-specific immunity on the part of the host. It has been described in a wide variety of protozoan species as indicated in Table 1. It has also been described in a number of bacterial species – *Neisseria gonnorhoeae*, *Borrelia hermsii*, *B. recurrentis*, *Anaplasma marginale*, and in the fungus, *Candida albicans* (Moxon *et al.* 1994; Donelson, 1995; Deitsch, Moxon & Wellems, 1997; Brayton *et al.* 2002). This wide phylogenetic distribution implies that it has evolved on multiple, independent occasions. The quality of the evidence differs considerably between pathogens, but this largely reflects the tractability of experimental analysis for any particular species.

It is interesting to note that 'antigenic' variation is not restricted to pathogens and has been described in two free-living species (Table 1). This observation is compelling evidence that clonal phenotypic variation can have a function other than to promote transmission and that the evolution of an infectious lifestyle does not necessarily predate the development of an ability to undergo this process. It is worth noting however, that both free-living species typically live in shallow freshwater habitats. An important variable in such habitats is temperature, changes in which lead to phenotypic variation in *Paramecium aurelia*. It is possible that phenotypic variation has a role in population survivorship in a capricious environment, analogous to that role of antigenic variation in parasites.

Comparing scenarios 1 and 2 in Fig. 1 could be construed as supporting a very traditional view in parasitology that 'a good parasite does not harm its host' (see for example Fantham & Porter, 1914) because it shows that evolution of a life history strategy by the pathogen that permits immune resolution of infection is of selective advantage to that pathogen. A comparison of scenarios 2 and 3 illustrates the fallacy of this view. Immune resolution of successive waves of pathogen population growth is essential to the success of antigenic variation as a transmission strategy, and yet chronic presence of the pathogen debilitates the host, lowering the lethality boundary (see Fig. 1). Clearly, this reduction of the boundary increases the possibility of it being breached as an infection progresses, but because an increased probability of host death is associated with improved transmission, harming the host can be of benefit to the pathogen.

Fig. 1 is an oversimplification of biological reality. It takes no account, for example, of the effects of co-infection either of different genotypes of the same species or of different species. It takes no account of the different courses of infection of zoonotic pathogens in different host species. The two boundaries (lethality and transmission) rarely represent simple step functions and trade-offs are to be expected between both probability of host death and transmission and between pathogen growth and transmission. Scenarios 2 and 3 envisage population size regulation by the immune response. However, regulation of growth rate, either by the pathogen itself or by the host, would be equally effective. All these factors would have evolutionary consequences that could impinge on the evolution of antigenic variation. Despite all these caveats, the essence of the link between antigenic variation and transmission remains, in my view, the most parsimonious explanation as to why phenotypic variation is of selective advantage to the host. However, I am not aware of any experimental evidence that *directly* tests this link and I fully accept that parsimony alone is insufficient reason to accept this hypothesis. This is a remarkable gap in the literature.

CONSERVED FEATURES OF ANTIGENIC VARIATION

A comparison of the mechanisms of antigenic variation in some of the organisms where it has been investigated supports the view of a polyphyletic origin for this process. At a superficial level there are shared features: reversible, mutually exclusive expression of members of gene family. But investigations of the mechanisms underlying antigenic variation reveal some stark contrasts. A good example of this contrast is the comparison of mechanisms of antigenic variation in the well studied prokaryotic and eukaryotic species, *Borrelia hermsii* and *Trypanosoma brucei*, respectively (Donelson, 1995).

If we take a functional rather than mechanistic perspective however, there is considerable similarity between systems used in different organisms. This similarity arises because there is, in my view, a restrictive set of five functional requirements that need to be met for antigenic variation to be of selective advantage to a parasite in evolutionary terms.

Firstly, a microorganism must have the capability to express several different antigens; minimally two. These variable antigens must be immunodominant over non-variable antigens, where the latter are defined as antigens that are identical in all cells in a clonal infection. 'Immunodominance' in this context indicates that functional immune responses to lower the numbers of pathogens (by killing them for instance) are directed preferentially to these antigens. Epitopes against which immune responses are generated must differ between variable antigens. The rate of switching between variable antigens per unit of time must be greater than the rate of immune clearance per unit of time.

Second, a microorganism must retain the capability to interact with its environment using non-variable antigens that must be immunologically 'silent' relative to variable antigens. To exploit the hosts' resources the parasite will need, for example, a glucose transporter to acquire glucose.

Third, individual cells within an infection must express variable antigens in a mutually exclusive manner. In the simplest scenario, if a cell expresses two variable antigens simultaneously, then the rate of immune clearance will be the same as if it had expressed only one of them. Thus the potential advantage of having the capability to express two variable antigens will have been lost.

Fourth, what applies to individual cells applies equally at the population level within an infection. Sub-populations, defined by their different variable antigens, must be expressed to minimise overlap in the timing of their expression (but see below).

Fifth, the pathogen must be capable of population growth within the mammalian host. For antigenic variation to occur successfully in the absence of growth, there would need to be a remarkable co-operativity between microorganisms to co-ordinate timing of switching and the order in which variable antigens were expressed. I find it difficult to conceive as to how such precise co-ordination could be initiated.

Taken together these five functional requirements give rise to four, 'cardinal signs' of antigenic variation – chronicity of infection, high rates of switching, hierarchical expression and reversible expression of variable antigens (Turner, 1999).

There are a number of issues that arise from these functional requirements and cardinal signs that should be highlighted in the context of evolution of antigenic variation. There will be a strong evolutionary drive towards divergence between variable antigens, at least for those epitopes that are immunodominant. This means that there is an expectation for much less sequence conservation between members of a gene family underlying antigenic variation than there would be for other gene families, potentially to the extent that identification of genes in any family using simple BLAST-based algorithms may fail. If there are regions or domains of genes that are conserved between family members this could be because of structural constraints on the proteins, lack of involvement in epitopes recognised by the immune system and/or because the proteins may combine a function for antigenic variation with a second function, such as cellular adhesion in malaria parasites.

There must, inevitably, be trade-offs between the first and second conserved features; variation and immunodominance versus conservation for interaction with the environment. It seems intuitively likely that such trade-offs would be important and interesting and yet they have been hardly explored from an evolutionary perspective. Indeed, I find it difficult to conceive of experimental approaches with the tools currently available in any protozoan parasite.

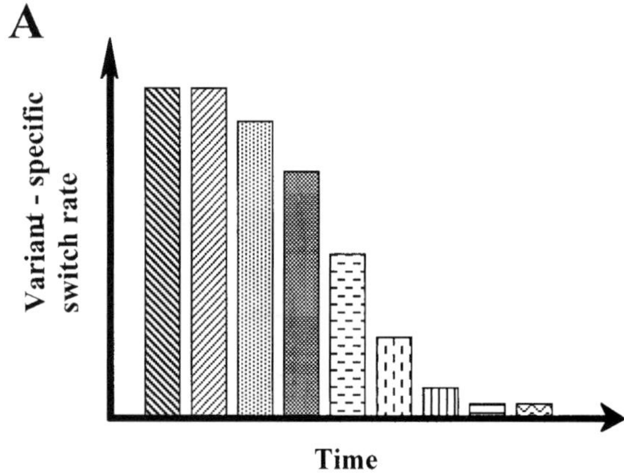

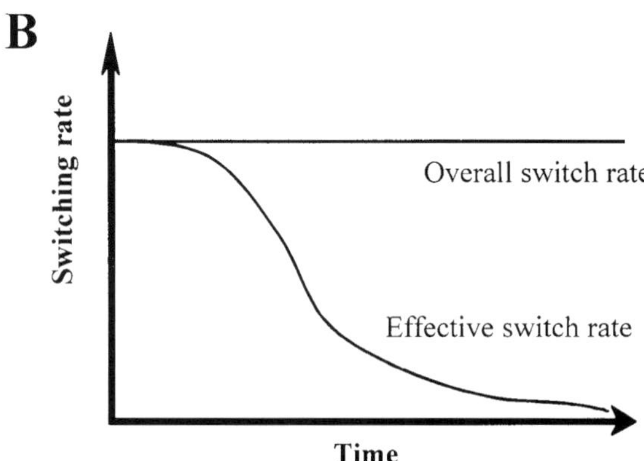

Fig. 2. A potential explanation of the relationship of hierarchical expression of variable antigens and the rate of antigenic switching. A. Switching between variable antigens is non-random and those that are switched to most frequently will appear first in an infection and generate variant-specific immune responses first. Thus there is predicted to be a negative correlation of VAT-specific switching rate and order of immune clearance. B. The effect of this is that, whilst the overall potential rate of antigenic variation remains high throughout an infection, in practice the effective rate of switching to expression of variants to which an immune response has not yet been generated will decline progressively.

ANTIGENIC SWITCHING – RATES, HIERARCHIES AND REVERSIBILITY

A more tractable line of enquiry has been the investigation of rates of antigenic switching. It seems self evident that the rate of switching must be higher than the immune response rate (when measured in equivalent units of time) although this statement does raise the issue that the latter does not appear to have been quantified for any host-pathogen system. It could be envisaged that, theoretically, a parasite might either modulate its switching rate in response to cues from the host or switch spontaneously at a high rate. In practice, all pathogens that have been studied in this respect appear to use the second approach, and they do so at remarkably high rates – typically greater than 1 in 1000 cells switches in each generation, two to four orders of magnitude higher than 'background' mutation rates (Turner, 1999).

I have previously argued that, for trypanosome infections, the very high rates of switching may have evolved as a bifunctional transmission-enhancing strategy that both evades and depresses immune responses (Turner, 1999). This possibility applies to the other parasites where multiple infections of hosts with isolates of overlapping variable antigen repertoires occur. Holoendemic malaria would be an excellent example of such a scenario. Competition between genotypes has the potential to lead to increased parasitaemia and higher switching rates. This result comes about because expression of a large variety of variable antigens at high levels will increase the potential to avoid any pre-existing immunity to some of those antigens and cross-immunity between variable antigens common to both genotypes. Any impairment of functional immunity is potentially of selective advantage to the parasite if it promotes transmission.

There is a trade-off required between causing immunodepression and evading immunity, and one way in which this might be managed is by hierarchical expression as illustrated in Fig. 2. Switching is non-random and those variable antigens that are

Table 2. Rates of switching between particular pairs of variable antigens differ, dependent on which antigen is being switched to. Data from Turner & Barry (1989) and Brannan *et al.* (1994). Switch rate values are switches/cell/generation for *T. brucei* and switches/schizont/generation for *P. chabaudi*; bld = below level of detection

Species	Expt.	Switch	Switch rate value
T. brucei	1	1·64 → 1·3	$2{\cdot}4 \times 10^{-3}$
		→ 1·22	$4{\cdot}0 \times 10^{-4}$
		→ 1·62	$1{\cdot}1 \times 10^{-4}$
	2	1·64 → 1·3	$6{\cdot}9 \times 10^{-3}$
		→ 1·22	$2{\cdot}2 \times 10^{-3}$
		→ 1.62	$1{\cdot}9 \times 10^{-6}$
P. chabaudi	1	Parent → RC4	$9{\cdot}2 \times 10^{-3}$
		→ RC10	$2{\cdot}9 \times 10^{-3}$
		→ RC7	$4{\cdot}3 \times 10^{-4}$
	2	Parent → RC4	$1{\cdot}3 \times 10^{-2}$
		→ RC10	$4{\cdot}0 \times 10^{-3}$
		→ RC7	bld

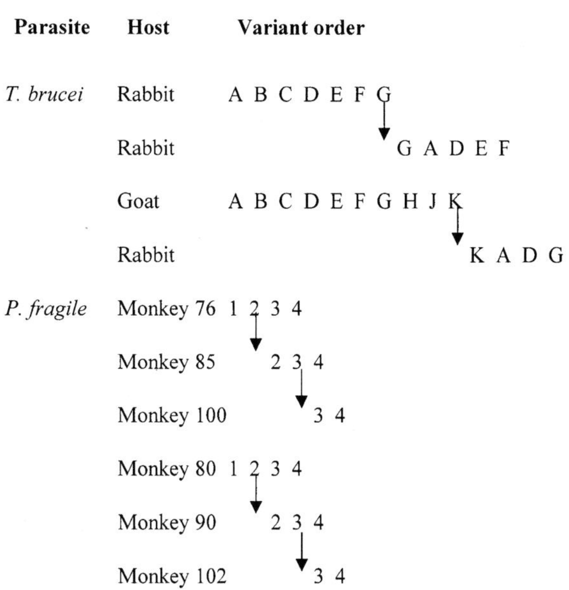

Fig. 3. Hierarchical expression and reversion of variant antigen expression compared in *T. brucei* and *P. fragile*. ↓, indicates transfer of parasites between hosts. There is hierarchical expression in both species leading to variant antigens being expressed in sequence in an infection. In *T. brucei* the hierarchy is 'reset' each time parasites are transferred to a new host thus demonstrating reversion of expression, but in *P. fragile* the hierarchy is not reset. Reversion has been demonstrated by other means (see text). Data derived from Gray (1965) and Handunetti *et al.* (1987). Not all variant antigens were sampled in the recipient hosts infected with *T. brucei*.

switched to most frequently will achieve highest prevalence earliest in an infection. These early variants will engender variant-specific immunity first and be eliminated leading to an inverse correlation of variant-specific switch rates and order of elimination. Because switching is a reversible process, there will continue to be many switch events later in infections back to expressions of variants against which effective immune responses are already in place and thus these switches will never be detected. In other words, there is massive redundancy in the system leading to progressively increasing numbers of suicide switch events and a concomitant reduction in the effective rate of switching which is the overall rate minus the suicide switches. The explanation shown in Fig. 2 would potentially explain mutually exclusive expression in pathogen populations (the fourth functional requirement in the previous section).

Very few studies have investigated hierarchical rates of switching, as opposed to hierarchical (non-random) expression of variants in an infection. What evidence there is (Table 2) supports the notion of hierarchical switch rates. The *per capita* values for switching rates may differ between replicate experiments for each species, but the patterns are consistent.

Fig. 3 illustrates an important distinction in hierarchical expression of variable antigens between *T. brucei* and *P. fragile*. In African trypanosomes, reversion of expression is observed *in vivo* when parasites are transferred between hosts as shown. The linear hierarchy is 'reset' for each new infection. [It is also not usually quite as predictable as shown in this particular example (Kosinski, 1980).] Such reversion has been detected in other parasites such as *G. lamblia* in *in vitro* culture (Nash, Conrad & Merrit, 1990). In *P. fragile* infections however, the hierarchy is *not* reset in each new host. *In vivo* data for *P. chabaudi* and *P. falciparum* also indicate no resetting of the hierarchy (MacLean, Pearson & Phillips, 1982; Hommel *et al.* 1991). Reversion of expression has been shown by other routes – in *in vitro* culture under positive selection for *P. falciparum* (by panning using a variant-specific antibody, Roberts *et al.* 1992), after mosquito transmission for *P. chabaudi* (MacLean *et al.* 1987) and by passaging of *P. fragile* in splenectomised monkeys (Handunetti, Mendis & David, 1987). There may be a fundamental distinction therefore between switching in parasites such as trypanosomes and *G. lamblia* on the one hand and *Plasmodium* spp. on the other. The explanation of hierarchical expression shown in Fig. 2 could apply to the former but not to the latter.

The important conclusion from this comparison is that the data on reversion of variable antigen expression in *Plasmodium* needs strengthening. The *in vivo* evidence for non-reversion in *P. falciparum* is based on a single experiment (Hommel *et al.* 1991), as is the *in vitro* demonstration of reversion (Roberts *et al.* 1992). The *in vivo* data are supported by the evidence from two other species. Reversion does not appear to have been investigated in *P. vivax* (del Portillo *et al.* 2001), or in the phylogenetically related parasite, *B. bovis* (Alred, 1998).

PERSPECTIVE

I have focused on (1) the link between antigenic variation and transmission, (2) the high rates of switching and (3) on hierarchical expression to illustrate that we know remarkably little as to how and why these work the way they do despite being, in my view, aspects of the process that are central to our understanding of antigenic variation. Experimental testing of (1), the hypothesis linking antigenic variation and transmission, is sorely needed. Underlying (2) and (3) is the issue of mutually exclusive expression. The explanation I offer above may be a partial answer in terms of the within-host population biology of an infection for some pathogens. For other pathogens it may not, although hopefully the observation may help direct future studies more appropriately. At the level of the single cell, we do not understand how mutually exclusive expression is regulated in any protozoan parasite that I am aware of. This is despite the best efforts of many very talented colleagues. Addressing these issues experimentally is extremely difficult work to undertake but it is essential because antigenic variation is such an important determinant of virulence in several major pathogens. Surely a stronger input from evolutionary biologists could only help?

ACKNOWLEDGEMENTS

I am grateful to The Wellcome Trust for financial support of my research.

REFERENCES

AL-KHEDERY, B., BARNWELL, J. W. & GALINSKI, M. R. (1999). Antigenic variation in malaria: a 3′ genomic alteration associated with the expression of *P. knowlesi* variant antigen. *Molecular Cell* **3**, 131–141.

ALRED, D. R. (1998). Antigenic variation in *Babesia bovis*: how similar is it to that in *Plasmodium falciparum*? *Annals of Tropical Medicine and Parasitology* **92**, 461–472.

ALRED, D. R., CARLTON, J. M. R., SATCHER, R. L., LONG, J. A., BROWN, W. C., PATTERSON, P. E., O'CONNOR, R. M. & STROUP, S. E. (2000). The *ves* multigene family of *B. bovis* encodes components of rapid antigenic variation at the infected erythrocyte surface. *Molecular Cell* **5**, 153–162.

BARRY, J. D. (1986). Antigenic variation during *Trypanosoma vivax* infections of different host species. *Parasitology* **92**, 51–65.

BARRY, J. D. & MCCULLOCH, R. (2001). Antigenic variation in Trypanosomes: Enhanced phenotypic variation in a eukaryotic parasite. *Advances in Parasitology* **49**, 1–70.

BRANNAN, L. R., TURNER, C. M. R. & PHILLIPS, R. S. (1994). Malaria parasites undergo antigenic variation at high rates *in vivo*. *Proceedings of the Royal Society London B* **256**, 71–75.

BRAYTON, K. A., PALMER, G. H., LUNDGREN, A., YI, J. & BARBET, F. (2002). Antigenic variation of *Anaplasma marginale msp2* occurs by combinatorial gene conversion. *Molecular Microbiology* **43**, 1151–1159.

BORST, P., BITTER, W., BLUNDELL, P. A., CHAVES, I., CROSS, M., GERRITS, H., VAN LEUVEN, F., MCCULLOUGH, R., TAYLOR, M. & RUDENKO, G. (1998). Control of VSG gene expression sites in *Trypanosoma brucei*. *Molecular and Biochemical Parasitology* **91**, 67–76.

CARON, F. & MEYER, E. (1989). Molecular basis of surface antigen variation in paramecia. *Annual Reviews of Microbiology* **43**, 23–42.

CRAIG, A. & SCHERF, A. (2001). Molecules on the surface of the *Plasmodium falciparum* infected erythrocyte and their role in malaria pathogenesis and immune evasion. *Molecular and Biochemical Parasitology* **115**, 129–143.

CROSS, G. A. M., WIRTZ, L. E. & NAVARRO, M. (1998). Regulation of VSG expression site transcription and switching in *Trypanosoma brucei*. *Molecular and Biochemical Parasitology* **91**, 77–91.

DEITSCH, K. W., MOXON, E. R. & WELLEMS, T. E. (1997). Shared themes of antigenic variation and virulence in bacterial, protozoal and fungal infections. *Microbiology and Molecular Biology Reviews* **61**, 281–293.

DEL PORTILLO, H. A., FERNANDEZ-BECERRA, C., BOWMAN, S., OLIVER, K., PREUSS, M., SANCHEZ, C. P., SCHNEIDER, N. K., VILLALOBOS, J. M., RAJANDREAM, M.-A., HARRIS, D., PEREIRA DA SILVA, L., BARRELL, B. & LANZER, M. (2001). A superfamily of variant genes encoded in the subtelomeric region of *Plasmodium vivax*. *Nature* **410**, 839–842.

DONELSON, J. E. (1995). Mechanisms of antigenic variation in *Borrelia hermsii* and African Trypanosomes. *Journal of Biological Chemistry* **270**, 7783–7786.

FANTHAM, H. B. & PORTER, A. (1914). *Some Minute Animal Parasites*. London, Methuen & Co.

GRAY, A. R. (1965). Antigenic variation in a strain of *Trypanosoma brucei* transmitted by *Glossina morsitans* and *G. palpalis*. *Journal of General Microbiology* **41**, 195–214.

HANDUNETTI, S. M., MENDIS, K. N. & DAVID, P. H. (1987). Antigenic variation of cloned *Plasmodium fragile* in its natural host *Macaca sinica*. *Journal of Experimental Medicine* **165**, 1269–1282.

HOMMEL, M., HUGHES, M., BOND, P. & CRAMPTON, J. M. (1991). Antibodies and DNA probes used to analyse variant populations of the Indochina-1 strain of *Plasmodium falciparum*. *Infection and Immunity* **59**, 3975–3981.

JONES, T. W. & MCKINNELL, C. D. (1985). Antigenic variation in *Trypanosoma evansi*; variable antigen type development in mice, sheep and goats. *Tropical Medicine and Parasitology* **36**, 53–57.

KOSINSKI, R. J. (1980). Antigenic variation in trypanosomes: a computer analysis of variant order. *Parasitology* **80**, 343–357.

MASAKE, R. A., MUSOKE, A. J. & NANTULYA, V. M. (1983). Specific antibody responses to the variable surface glycoprotein of *Trypanosoma congolense* in infected cattle. *Parasite Immunology* **5**, 345–355.

MCLEAN, S. A., PEARSON, C. D. & PHILLIPS, R. S. (1982). *Plasmodium chabaudi*: Antigenic variation during recrudescent parasitaemias in mice. *Experimental Parasitology* **54**, 296–302.

McLEAN, S. A., PHILLIPS, R. S., PEARSON, C. D. & WALLIKER, D. (1987). The effect of mosquito transmission of antigenic variants of *Plasmodium chabaudi*. *Parasitology* **94**, 443–449.

MOXON, E. R., RAINEY, P. B., NOWAK, M. A. & LENSKI, R. E. (1994). Adaptive evolution of highly mutable loci in pathogenic bacteria. *Current Biology* **4**, 24–33.

NASH, T. E., CONRAD, J. T. & MERRIT, JR., J. W. (1990). Variant specific epitopes of *Giardia lamblia*. *Molecular and Biochemical Parasitology* **42**, 125–132.

PAYS, E. & NOLAN, D. P. (1998). Expression and function of surface proteins in *Trypanosoma brucei*. *Molecular and Biochemical Parasitology* **91**, 3–36.

PHILLIPS, R. S., BRANNAN, L. R., BALMER, P. & NEUVILLE, P. (1997). Antigenic variation during malaria infection – the contribution from the murine parasite *Plasmodium chabaudi*. *Parasite Immunology* **19**, 427–434.

PREER, J. R. (1986). Surface antigens of *Paramecium*. In *The Molecular Biology of Ciliated Protozoa* (ed. J. G. Gull), pp. 301–339. New York, Academic Press

ROBERTS, D. J., CRAIG, A. G., BERENDT, A. R., PINCHES, R., NAHS, G., MARSH, K. & NEWBOLD, C. I. (1992). Rapid switching to multiple antigenic and adhesive phenotypes in malaria. *Nature* **357**, 689–692.

SVÄRD, S. G., MENG, T., HETSKO, M. L., McCAFFERY, J. M. & GILLIN, F. D. (1998). Differentiation-associated surface antigen variation in the ancient eukaryote *Gardia lamblia*. *Molecular Microbiology* **30**, 979–989.

TURNER, C. M. R. (1999). Antigenic variation in *Trypanosoma brucei* infections: a holistic view. *Journal of Cell Science* **112**, 3187–3912.

TURNER, C. M. R. & BARRY, J. D. (1989). High frequency of antigenic variation in *Trypanosoma brucei rhodesiense* infections. *Parasitology* **99**, 67–75.

Variation and polymorphism in helminth parasites

R. M. MAIZELS[1]* *and* A. KURNIAWAN-ATMADJA[2]

[1] *Institute of Cell, Animal and Population Biology, University of Edinburgh, West Mains Road, Edinburgh EH9 3JT, UK*
[2] *Department of Parasitology, Faculty of Medicine, University of Indonesia, Salemba Raya 6, Jakarta 10430, Indonesia*

SUMMARY

There are strong biological, evolutionary and immunological arguments for predicting extensive polymorphism among helminth parasites, but relatively little data and few instances from which the selective forces acting on parasite diversity can be discerned. The paucity of information on intraspecific variation stands in contrast to the fine detail with which helminth species have been delineated by morphological techniques, accentuating a trend towards considering laboratory strains as representative of a relatively invariant organism. However, in the fast-moving evolutionary race between host and parasite one would predict a monomorphic species would be driven to extinction. We review the arena of intraspecific variation for the major helminth parasites, ranging from biological properties such as host or vector preference, to biochemical and immunological characteristics, as well as molecular markers such as DNA sequence variants. These data are summarized, before focusing in more detail on polymorphisms within protein-coding genes of potential relevance to the host-parasite relationship, such as vaccine candidates. In particular, we discuss the available data on a number of major antigens from the filarial nematode *Brugia malayi*. Information is currently too sparse to answer the question of whether there is antigenic variation in filariasis, but the indications are that proteins from the blood-borne microfilarial stage show significant intraspecific variability. Future work will define whether polymorphisms in these antigens may be driven by exposure to the host immune response or reflect some other facet of parasite biology.

Key words: Antigenic variation, genetic polymorphism, nematodes, filariasis.

INTRODUCTION

As we proceed in this exciting era of genome sequencing, unwrapping details of thousands of new genes from pathogens large and small, it is becoming increasingly obvious that information from a single 'type' individual will not suffice. The complete genome sequence of any organism is indeed the gateway to the functional biology of novel genes, identification of new drug targets and vaccine antigens, and in establishing the fundamental physiology of highly evolved parasites with specialized lifestyles (Blaxter *et al.* 1999; Johnston *et al.* 1999). Here however, we wish to review where we stand on the question of polymorphism of helminth parasites, with the perspective that a genome sequence represents but one reference point against which many variant sequence types may be found within the same species. Within this context, our focus will be on protein-coding sequences, genes for functional proteins in which allelic variation may act to modify biological activity, or provide diversity in the face of specific host immune responses. Such analyses are conspicuously rare for any helminth parasite (Read & Viney, 1996).

The study of helminth protein polymorphisms has been hindered by three issues. First, there is the biological problem that helminth parasites are, in general, sexually reproducing animals which do not themselves multiply in their host. Thus clonal populations do not exist (except in a few circumscribed instances), requiring that the analysis of coding alleles be performed on individual worms. Second, in many species the quantities of protein (or even DNA) that can be recovered from one individual precludes many analyses. Thirdly, where field isolates require propagation through laboratory animals, it is likely that this very propagation reduces the variability in the parasite by selecting subpopulations best adapted to the unnatural host (LoVerde *et al.* 1985; Curtis & Minchella, 2000).

Why then should we study 'wild' helminths? There are both practical and theoretical imperatives to do so. The development of vaccine candidate antigens cannot proceed far without knowledge of the distribution and conservation of antigen genes among parasite populations worldwide. Moreover, the critical question of whether helminth parasites display any form of antigenic variation has not been systematically addressed despite the fundamental implications this would have on the whole of parasite immunology.

Equally important is the threat posed by drug-resistance alleles to the success of basic anthelmintic therapy (Sangster, 1996; Prichard, 2001). Conceptually, we need to understand the population genetic structure of helminth parasites to predict how such resistance alleles may spread and reach fixation in natural populations. This requires more data on allele frequency, interbreeding and molecular variation among all important helminth species (Nadler,

* To whom correspondence should be addressed. Phone: (+44) 131-650-5511. Fax: (+44) 131-650-5450. E-mail: r.maizels@ed.ac.uk

DOI: 10.1017/S0031182002001890 Printed in the United Kingdom

1995; Anderson, Blouin & Beech, 1998). In addition, there is the argument that natural variation in genes provides a spotlight on proteins with interesting functions in the host-parasite relationship. Furthermore, comparisons between isogenic organisms differing at only one locus can provide a far more conclusive link between gene and function than any number of analyses of newly-identified sequences in a single isolate.

In this review, we discuss the currently known polymorphisms in helminths generally, and then proceed to consider the filarial nematodes in particular. We illustrate this with examples from the literature and from our own recent work in Indonesia.

HELMINTH POLYMORPHISM

There are plenty of documented polymorphisms for helminth parasites, whether judged by biological characteristics (e.g. morphology, infectivity), biochemical (e.g. enzymatic and susceptibility to anthelmintic drugs), immunological (e.g. antibody reactivity) or molecular biological (e.g. DNA sequence) (McManus & Bowles, 1996; Read & Viney, 1996; Wakelin & Goyal, 1996). We discuss each of these issues briefly below.

Most contemporary molecular information involves non-coding sequences such as microsatellite dinucleotide repeats and spacing regions flanking mitochondrial genes. This field has been recently reviewed by Anderson *et al.* (1998) and so will not be discussed in detail here. A good example of the potential of these marker sequences is in Anderson's own work describing the separate population structures of human and swine *Ascaris* parasites in the Americas (Anderson, Romero-Abal & Jaenike, 1993; 1995). In a different manner, a particularly interesting sequence variation has emerged from *Haemonchus contortus* in which the random interpolation of a short transposable sequence has been noted (Hoekstra *et al.* 2000). These variants appear to have little functional consequence, but have proven invaluable markers to identify 'strains' and geographical isolates of the parasite.

INFECTIVITY AND SURVIVAL IN THE HOST

Infectivity is perhaps the characteristic of most intrinsic importance to parasites, and has been carefully studied in most major species. Not only is there a great practical importance to knowing which parasite types may be most infective to target species, but variation in infectivity patterns can give insights into how the infection process itself is controlled. Several examples can be drawn from nematode parasites of humans and animals. Different isolates of the gastrointestinal nematode *Trichuris muris* vary in their ability to resist immune-mediated expulsion by mice (Bellaby *et al.* 1995). Parasite survival appears to be associated with the type of immune response stimulated in the host, as the most persistent isolate induces a stronger 'Th1' bias than the others (Bellaby, Robinson & Wakelin, 1996). The Th1 response is pro-inflammatory, typically through macrophage activation, and while well-adapted to eliminating intracellular micro-organisms is known to be ineffective against nematode parasites in the gut. Significantly, sharp differences in infectivity can be observed in sibling lines of *T. muris* derived from a single isolate, indicating that the parasite population in the wild is polymorphic in this respect (as described elsewhere in this supplement by D. Wakelin *et al.*). Similarly, *Trichinella* parasites from various geographical locales show markedly different infectivities to laboratory mice, as well as differences in the extent to which they elicit a protective 'Th2' immune response (Bolas-Fernandez & Wakelin, 1990; Wakelin & Goyal, 1996).

Many helminth parasites can be 'adapted' to laboratory animal species which are not their natural hosts. For example, *Necator americanus*, a human hookworm, can be 'adapted' to hamsters (Sen, 1972) and laboratory rat strains of *Nippostrongylus brasiliensis* to optimal infection of mice (Solomon & Haley, 1966; Wescott & Todd, 1966). A fascinating set of experiments were conducted by Dobson and coworkers, in which lines of *Heligmosomoides polygyrus* were propagated by serial passage through naive or immune mice, and the latter set of parasites shown to be less immunogenic (Su & Dobson, 1997). Similar selection experiments in other nematode species have had variable results (reviewed by Read & Viney, 1996), with adaptation evident after a single passage, or failing to be evident at all. A missing factor from these experiments is any genetic marker in order to establish that adaptation represents selection from a polymorphic ancestral population, and to exclude any heritable epigenetic mechanism.

A clearer indication that different host species select distinct subpopulations of parasites comes from studies on *Schistosoma mansoni*, (LoVerde *et al.* 1985). A single African isolate has been propagated separately for many years in baboons and mice. The baboon parasites are polymorphic at several loci, while single alleles have become fixed in the murine population. When baboon-derived parasites were 'adapted' by serial passage in mice, the resultant parasites were found to have fixed the same alleles as in the original mouse strain, indicating selective pressure against certain alleles is exerted in the mouse environment.

BIOCHEMICAL VARIATION

Biochemical polymorphisms are evident from almost all isoenzyme (or allozyme) analyses (Anderson *et al.* 1998), but their use in determining an average level of parasite genetic variability has been interpreted in different ways. The mean heterozygosity in any one individual *Ascaris* was found to be only 2 of 38 loci (6·6 %), leading to the suggestion that gastrointestinal parasites were relatively monomorphic (Leslie *et al.* 1982). However, in other closely related ascarid worms such as *Toxocara*, Nadler (1986) found a much higher level (8·5–13·7 %) mean heterozygosity, and reported that 22–39 % of all loci tested showed some degree of allelic polymorphism across the population as a whole. These data led Nadler (1990) to reach a contrary conclusion, that ascarids do display considerable genetic diversity. Another proposal was that nematodes with direct life cycles were less polymorphic than those with indirect life histories, but again this association was not supported by an analysis of data from some 35 nematode species (Anderson *et al.* 1998). With expressed sequence tag (EST) data from many of these species now identifying the enzymes in question at the sequence level, it would be both possible and timely to quantify the heterozygosity and degree of sequence variation in these same enzymes to resolve these questions.

An example of the more precise information now available in the biochemical arena is the identification of alleles responsible for drug resistance in nematodes. Benzimidazole resistance in gastrointestinal nematodes of pastoral animals, a phenomenon of considerable concern (Sangster, 1996), can be attributed to 2 specific amino acid substitutions in the β-tubulin protein, which itself is encoded at two separate loci. The predominant susceptible allele encodes Tyr-200, and the resistant allele Phe-200, in both *H. contortus* (Kwa, Veenstra & Roos, 1994) and *Teladorsagia circumcincta* (Elard, Comes & Humbert, 1996). Moreover, resistance is enhanced if Phe-167 changes to Tyr or His (Prichard, 2001), and increasing degrees of resistance occur when these substitutions coincide, when they are present at both loci, and when either or both loci become homozygous for a resistance allele. The rapidity with which drug selection appears indicates that the resistant alleles are pre-existing in the wild populations.

An even greater degree of polymorphism is observed in the P-glycoprotein gene of *H. contortus*, thought to be important in multi-drug resistance (Blackhall *et al.* 1998). No fewer than 7 alleles, defined by restriction fragment length polymorphism, were found in just 30 individual worms from a single strain. A larger comparison of 5 different strains (3 of which had been selected through 17 generations of ivermectin- and moxidectin-treated sheep infection) identified some 31 RFLP alleles in a total of 180 individuals. Although individual alleles were not sequenced, this system perhaps represents the most polymorphic yet described for any helminth gene.

IMMUNOLOGICAL VARIATION

Immunological variation within individual helminth species has been the most elusive to identify at the genetic level. One may expect that the ceaseless 'arms race' between host and parasite has generated a wide variety of antigenic variants, but no conclusive evidence has yet been provided. One direct approach to this question is to screen parasite populations with specific antibodies. *Ascaris* larvae do vary in surface binding to human antibody, but this may be phenotypic as different individual worms could express quantitatively different levels of surface antigens, or may be out of phase in development (Fraser & Kennedy, 1991). Gilleard described a monoclonal antibody, generated to *Dictyocaulus viviparus*, which binds only to a subpopulation of *Necator americanus* larvae (Gilleard, Duncan & Tait, 1995). As with *Ascaris*, this enticing observation has yet to be linked to an inherited factor within the parasite population. If substantiated, such instances would have direct relevance to immune system recognition, immunity and parasite immune evasion mechanisms.

Some studies have addressed the critical question of whether vaccines and vaccine antigens from different isolates are equally efficacious. Irradiated cercariae of *S. mansoni* induce partial protection against subsequent challenge with undamaged parasites. When mice were vaccinated with irradiated *S. mansoni* from Egypt or Puerto Rico, the protection against the homologous isolate was broadly similar, but cross-protection was not reciprocal (Hackett *et al.* 1987). In *S. japonicum*, a Chinese isolate propagated in the laboratory since 1937 immunized effectively against challenge with 3 wild isolates taken 50 years later (Moloney, Hinchcliffe & Webbe, 1989), but failed to protect against a Phillipine strain (Moloney, Garcia & Webbe, 1985). In the case of *Trichinella spiralis*, isolates from Spain, Poland and London showed variable levels of protective immunization when tested against homologous challenge, but markedly poorer protection against heterologous infection in some combinations (Goyal & Wakelin, 1993). At the very least, antigens involved in protective immunity do not appear to be fully conserved within species. Studies such as these place greater urgency on defining the precise structural polymorphisms at the amino acid sequence level. As argued elsewhere, if vaccine antigen targets are in fact highly variable, this brings into question the utility of those antigens which may be so effective in the laboratory context.

POLYMORPHISMS IN CODING SEQUENCES

A number of recent studies have explicitly sought intraspecific comparisons between potential alleles of

Table 1. Sequence polymorphisms in coding genes of nematode parasites

Species	Comparison	Gene	aa variation	nt variation	Reference
Ancylostoma caninum	China vs US isolates	ASP-1 (VAL-1)	10/424	42/1271	(Qiang *et al.* 2000)
Brugia malayi	TRS strain	ALT-2	0/128	137 nt in intron	(Gregory *et al.* 2000)
	TRS strain	CPI-2	1/161	1/483	(Gregory & Maizels, unpublished)
	Indonesia isolates	SHP-1	6/205	12/615	Kurniawan-Atmadja *et al.* unpublished
	Indonesia isolates	SHP-5	5/161	9/632	Kurniawan-Atmadja *et al.* unpublished
	TRS strain	VAL-1	0/220	2/660	(Murray *et al.* 2001)
Haemonchus contortus	Benzimidazole (BZ) resistant vs susceptible	β-tubulin isotypes I and/or II	4/448	na	(Beech *et al.* 1994); (Kwa *et al.* 1994)
Onchocerca volvulus	Blinding vs non-blinding	PDI	0/281	1/843	(Keddie *et al.* 1999)
	Blinding vs non-blinding	CAR	0/337	0/1011	(Keddie *et al.* 1999)
	Blinding vs non-blinding	API	0/240	0/720	(Keddie *et al.* 1999)
	Blinding vs non-blinding	RAL2	0/140	0/420	(Keddie *et al.* 1999)
	Mali vs Cameroon	Actin-2	1/376	1/1125	(Zeng & Donelson, 1992)
Teladorsagia circumcincta	BZ resistant vs susceptible	β-tubulin isotype I	1/371	na	(Elard *et al.* 1996)

Ac-ASP-1 = *Ancylostoma* secreted protein-1.
Bm-ALT-2 = Abundant larval transcript-2. Polymorphism is in repeat motif of intron 3.
Bm-CPI-2 = Cysteine protease inhibitor-2. Polymorphism is aa 67 (Lys/Asn).
Bm-SHP-1, SHP-5 = Sheath protein-1, -5 of the microfilarial sheath. Preliminary data are cited. Multiple deletion events (5-aa in SHP-1 and 8-aa in SHP-5) are counted as a single difference.
Bm-VAL-1 = Vespid venom, *Ancylostoma* secreted protein-Like-1. Polymorphisms at nt 219 and 351 of ORF are synonymous.
Hc-β-tubulin: there are two loci, each of which can contribute to benzimidazole resistance. When both loci are homozygous for a resistant allele, worms are highly resistant. Resistant alleles may have substitutions at either or both 167 (Phe/Tyr or His) and 200 (Phe/Tyr) (Prichard, 2001). Additionally residues 76 and 368 have been reported to differ between resistant and susceptible isolates (Kwa *et al.* 1994).
Ov-Actin-2. Polymorphism at aa 205 (Ala/Val).
Tc-β-tubulin. Polymorphism at aa 200 (Phe/Tyr). Data obtained only on aa 60-430.

coding genes (Table 1). One investigation focused on a candidate vaccine antigen from hookworm, termed *Ancylostoma* secreted protein (ASP) (Hawdon *et al.* 1996). ASP belongs to a large gene family represented in all nematodes so far studied, and with more distant relatives in all other taxa from plants to mammals. When *Ancylostoma caninum* samples derived from dogs in China and the USA were compared (Qiang *et al.* 2000), 10 amino acid substitutions were found in the 421-amino acid protein (2 of the changes being within the short N-terminal signal sequence); this is a relatively low level of diversity, and the applicability of ASP-1 for vaccination is promising as one domain of the protein showed only one amino acid difference. At the nucleotide level, there were a total of 30 nucleotide changes in ~1300 bp, the ratio of coding to non-coding changes implying that all may be neutral.

It surely is essential that similar studies are undertaken on vaccine candidate antigens for other major helminth parasites. The paucity of species-wide data on sequence diversity or conservation of the antigens selected for development as schistosomiasis vaccine components has been commented upon elsewhere (Curtis & Minchella, 2000). One wonders whether an approach which identifies the most variable antigens across the species as a whole should not be a mandatory part of the vaccine development process?

While studies such as these deal with protein coding sequence allelisms, it is important to remember that many functional polymorphisms are coded in regulatory elements within non-coding DNA (e.g. promoter and enhancer sequences), in RNA elements, and within introns of protein-coding genes. Analyses of these regions is likely to receive more attention once individual proteins of known importance are analysed in sufficient detail.

FILARIASIS: BIOLOGICAL DIVERSITY

Lymphatic filariasis is primarily caused by two closely related nematodes, *Brugia malayi* and *Wuchereria bancrofti*. The microfilarial (Mf) stages of *B. malayi* and *W. bancrofti* can be distinguished by the cell nuclei at the caudal tip visible in the former species, and adults differ in details of external morphology, such as the numbers of papillae. The principal distinction is size, the adults of *W. bancrofti* reaching a maximum about 50% larger than *B. malayi*. Although these may appear slender grounds for separation of *B. malayi* into a distinct genus (Buckley, 1960), it is generally felt that any further change in nomenclature would not serve the field well.

In addition to these two major species, there are additional members of each genus. The human parasite *B. timori* has a restricted distribution but causes disease very similar to *B. malayi*. The animal filaria *B. pahangi* is considered non-infective to humans, but is known to form fertile hybrids with *B. malayi*. These three *Brugia* species show extensive antigenic similarities (Maizels *et al.* 1983). There are at least 6 additional species of *Brugia* (Sasa, 1976), and one other known species of *Wuchereria* (*W. kalimantani*), found in the silvered leaf monkey *Presbytis cristatus* (Palmieri *et al.* 1980).

Within individual species, it is known that the adult male worms of *B. malayi* show significant morphological variation with respect to their posterior cuticular ornamentation (required for successful mating), and these features distinguish isolates from China, India, Indonesia/Malaysia and Korea (Bain *et al.* 1989). However, the most striking variation within the species of both *B. malayi* and *W. bancrofti* are those observed with respect to periodicity. This remarkable feature describes the circadian rhythm with which microfilarial numbers rise and fall in the peripheral blood, in apparent synchrony with the biting behaviour of the local mosquito species (Hawking, 1975). Most *W. bancrofti* infections are nocturnally periodic, with few Mf present in the peripheral blood during the daytime hours. Exceptionally, the Pacific variant is diurnally periodic in accordance with the daytime biting habits of the *Aedes* mosquitoes.

B. malayi shows a wider variety of periodicities, but most parasites are either nocturnally periodic or sub-periodic, a dichotomy within the species which was established by Wilson *et al.* in 1959. These authors reported that periodic *B. malayi* was typically *Anopheles*-transmitted, rarely found in animals, and had slightly longer Mf which typically cast their sheath when stained with Giemsa on a thin blood film. In contrast, the subperiodic parasites were generally *Mansonia*-transmitted, could be found naturally in, and readily transmitted to, cats, and had Mf which retained their sheath on Giemsa staining. This subdivision into periodic and sub-periodic is often still followed in the filariasis literature.

The question of periodicity and subdivision of *B. malayi* into biological types was thoroughly re-examined by Partono & Purnomo (1987). They identified several problems. First, periodicity indices (e.g. the ratio of night-time peak to the daytime nadir) drew an arbitrary borderline between the 'periodic' and 'subperiodic' types. Second, some isolates (e.g. East Kalimantan) were in fact aperiodic, although in all other respects such as infectivity to non-human hosts were like the subperiodic. Third, and most importantly, isolates such as Pekan Baru showed nocturnal periodicity but were otherwise 'subperiodic' with features such as *Mansonia* transmission and infectivity to laboratory animals. Reviewing the biological properties of some 10 isolates from diverse localities in Indonesia, Partono and Purnomo concluded that the key differentiating factor was infectivity to animals, thus reclassifying the 'periodic' type as anthropophilic and the 'subperiodic' as zoophilic. This revised division is one we endorse and, presenting it in Table 2, we suggest that it becomes the standard nomenclature.

Most *B. malayi* across South and East Asia is the periodic or anthropophilic type, while the zoophilic type is restricted to Indonesia, Malaysia and the Phillipines (Sasa, 1976). A variant of the anthrophilic type, termed the rocky beach strain, was described as being *Aedes*-transmitted in Korea and Japan, but has not been further characterized (Sasa, 1976). The strain of *B. malayi* used in most laboratories is a zoophilic type, originating in Pahang in West Malaysia (Edeson & Wharton, 1958). This strain is now propagated by TRS Labs Inc. of Georgia, USA, after which the strain is named. There is no explicit indication of any differential pathology between the different strains of *B. malayi*, in the manner distinguishing Bancroftian filariasis from the Brugian form of the disease (Partono, 1987).

Molecular polymorphisms among the *B. malayi* strains have been demonstrated by Underwood *et al.* (2000) using two microsatellite markers. BMsat1 shows that several zoophilic isolates from Indonesia have a microsatellite allele which is 2 bp longer than the allele from the one anthropophilic parasite tested, and 2 bp shorter than the allele present in the TRS strain. One Indonesian isolate also showed 6 bp longer form of the microsatellite BMsat2. Interestingly, this microsatellite is suggested to reside within a novel protein coding sequence, which is maintained in-frame by the 6 bp insertion.

FILARIASIS: ANTIGENIC DIVERSITY IN IMMUNOLOGICAL STUDIES

Antigenic variation or diversity is an evolutionary strategy for pathogens to escape the effects of a specific immune response mediated by, for example,

Table 2. Morphological and ecological variants of lymphatic filarial nematodes

Lymphatic Filariae	
Anthropophilic *B. malayi* Nocturnally periodic Mf exsheath Difficult to infect jirds (low microfilaraemia, short patency) Rice cultivation ecosystem *Anopheles barbirostris* vector No reservoir host China, India (Kerala), Indonesia (South and Central Sulawesi), Korea, Malaysia (Penang)	Zoophilic *B. malayi* Subperiodic, periodic or aperiodic Mf do not exsheath Easily infect jirds Swamp ecosystem *Mansonia* vector Reservoir hosts (monkeys, cats) Indonesia (Kalimantan, Buru, Tanjungpinang, Kendari, Pekan Baru, Bengkulu, Jambi, Lampung), Malaysia (Pahang) and Phillipines
Periodic *W. bancrofti* Nocturnally periodic *Culex* (urban) and *Anopheles/Aedes* (rural) No reservoir host Africa, Americas, Asia	*W. bancrofti* var *pacifica* Diurnally subperiodic, *Aedes* vector No reservoir host Polynesia
B. timori Nocturnally periodic *Anopheles barbirostris* vector No reservoir host Timor, Flores, Alor islands	

antibodies. Although the role of antibodies in human immunity is not established, there is an inverse relationship between detectable antibody binding to the surface of Mf, and the presence of Mf themselves (McGreevy *et al.* 1980) suggesting that antibodies mediate clearance of Mf. If so, then the antigens on the external sheath of Mf may be expected to vary within one filarial species.

Whether Mf surface antigens do indeed vary has been directly addressed in only one study (Ravindran, Satapathy & Sahoo, 1994). Stimulated by the observation that around 20% of Mf+ individuals do have antibodies that bind to the surface of Mf, and that in all published assays the Mf used for testing were taken from a heterologous individual, these authors collected parasites and sera from 5 Mf+ patients. None of the patients' sera reacted to their own (autologous) Mf, although one showed fluorescent binding to heterologous Mf. When a panel of unrelated patient sera was tested against these 5 isolates of Mf, all elephantiasis sera reacted to all isolates. Most significantly, of sera from 15 additional Mf+ patients, no fewer than 7 recognized one or more of the 5 test isolates from unrelated patients. These results suggest that Mf can express a variety of surface antigens, and that those that survive in the human bloodstream are those which the host antibody response fails to recognize.

The target antigens of this reaction have yet to be defined. The Mf sheath is composed of a tightly cross-linked set of repeat-rich proteins, together with some carbohydrate structures (Hirzmann *et al.* 1995; Zahner, Hobom & Stirm, 1995). The key proteins (SHP-1, -2, -3 and variants thereof) have all been defined, but the accessibility of antibodies to each protein on acetone-fixed Mf has not been established. Interestingly, Ravindran and colleagues found that antibody binding was not sensitive to protease treatment of the Mf. This does not necessarily indicate a carbohydrate target, as the dense cross-linking of sheath proteins is likely to protect them from proteolysis.

MOLECULAR POLYMORPHISMS IN FILARIAL ANTIGENS

Few systematic analyses have yet been carried out at the molecular level for variation of any filarial antigen, but interesting data have already emerged as a result of studies executed for other purposes. For example, the Filarial Genome Project has provided partial cDNA sequences from some 22,000 cDNA clones from *B. malayi* (The Filarial Genome Project, 1999). All these clones are derived from the TRS strain, and yet minor sequence variants representing putative alleles can be observed within this one dataset. These presumably correspond to polymorphisms which have survived repeated passage through laboratory animals. Another window available is to compare the pattern of evolutionary change in homologous molecules from related species (*B. malayi/B. pahangi* and *B. malayi/W. bancrofti*). We review below our current information drawn from these sources on selected filarial antigens; these antigens have been reviewed in more detail elsewhere (Maizels, Blaxter & Scott, 2001).

Table 3. Intron and exon variation in two filarial antigens

	B. malayi vs *B. pahangi*	*B. malayi* vs *W. bancrofti*
GPX-1/GP29		
Introns		
(n = 3, 949 nt)	88	199
Exons		
(n = 4, 669 nt)	7	17
(n = 4, 223 aa)	0	7
SHP-1/MF22		
Introns		
(n = 1, 78 nt)	2 (2·6 %)	
Exons		
Exon 1 (367 nt 122 aa)	19 nt	
	15 aa	
Exon 2 (248 nt 83 aa)	11 nt	
	5 aa	

Glutathione peroxidase (GPX-1)

The major surface protein in the cuticle of adult filarial parasite is a 29 kDa glycoprotein (Maizels *et al.* 1989) shown both by sequence analysis (Cookson, Blaxter & Selkirk, 1992) and functional characterization (Tang *et al.* 1996) to be the antioxidant enzyme glutathione peroxidase. The GPX-1 antigen is also strongly recognized by human antibodies, indicating that it could be under immune selection. By sequencing genomic copies of this gene from *B. pahangi*, *B. malayi* and *W. bancrofti* (Cookson, Tang & Selkirk, 1993), the analysis presented in Table 3 emerged. Remarkably, GPX-1 from the two *Brugia* species has identical amino acid sequence, with only 7/669 (1·0 %) synonymous nucleotide differences. The rate of nucleotide substitution in the introns (9·3 %) is nearly ten times higher than in the exons, in comparisons of the same two species. The complete conservation of coding sequence is more compatible with a strict functional constraint than with a model of immune evasion by antigen variation. Even when differences between *B. malayi* and *W. bancrofti* are considered, and coding changes become evident (3·1 %), the numbers of non-synonymous and synonymous nucleotide substitutions (7 and 10 respectively) do not support the hypothesis that variability of this antigen is driven by the host immune response.

Cysteine Protease Inhibitor-2 (CPI-2)

Another prominent surface and secreted product from adult filarial worms is a 15 kDa member of the cysteine protease inhibitor (cystatin) family (Gregory and Maizels, unpublished). Represented frequently in the EST database, sequences for CPI-2 display a dimorphism: approximately equal numbers have either lysine or asparagine at residue 89. No functional difference is apparent in terms of protease inhibition, and the residue is not involved in either of the two protease-reactive sites. However, the asparagine-encoding form provides a potential N-glycosylation site. Most interestingly, the same dimorphism is observed in the *Onchocerca volvulus* EST dataset.

Abundant Larval Transcript-2 (ALT-2)

A most intriguing set of L3-associated antigens in filarial nematodes is the Abundant Larval Transcript (ALT) family (Gregory *et al.* 2000; Maizels *et al.* 2001), which represent 1–10 % of cDNAs in various filarial species at the L3 stage, but are barely found at other points in the life cycle. They are the front-running candidates for vaccine antigens. So far, the family has been characterized by numerous related genes rather than variants at any one locus, and coding polymorphisms have yet to be identified. However, we have established that within the TRS laboratory strain, one of the ALT family (ALT-2) exhibits variant forms of intron 3. Intron 3 is itself unusual in consisting of a repeat sequence, and two forms of differing repeat numbers are found (Fig. 1). Individual worms possess either or both these forms, consistent with the notion that they are Mendelian alleles (W. F. Gregory & N. Gomez-Escobar, unpublished).

Another ALT family member is the dominant product from larvae of *Onchocerca* species (Bianco, Wu & Jenkins, 1995; Joseph, Huima & Lustigman, 1998). In a striking experiment, individual L3 of *O. lienalis* were labelled by injecting infected blackflies with radioactive methionine. The resulting analysis showed a size polymorphism in this protein taken from 11 individual parasites (Blanco *et al.* 1990). Thus, there are appear to be coding variants as well as intronic variants of this important gene family.

The significance of the intron dimorphism remains to be defined, but intronic alleles are known to affect levels of expression in *Drosophila* (Laurie & Stam, 1994; Stam & Laurie, 1996) as well as in higher

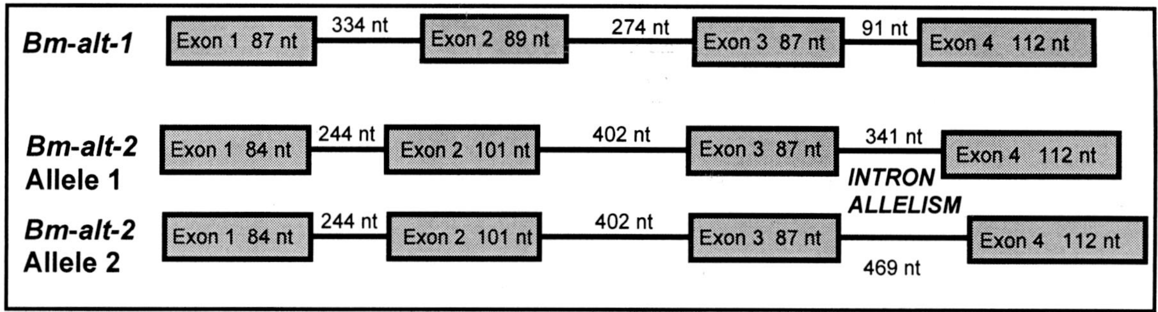

Fig. 1. Intron polymorphism in *B. malayi* abundant larval transcript-2 gene. Gene structures of *B. malayi alt-1* and *alt-2*, as described by Gregory *et al.* (2000) with further data on the 1st intron from unpublished data of Dr Natalia Gomez-Escobar (personal communication). Alleles shown are both represented in the TRS laboratory strain. Boxes represent exons, thin lines are introns with nucleotide lengths given. Not to scale.

animals. Generally, greater effects are attributed to substitutions in the first intron, where enhancer sequences are often positioned, but in other cases polymorphisms in repeat motifs of downstream introns can regulate levels of gene expression (Shimogiri *et al.* 1998; MacKenzie & Quinn, 1999). Allelic diversity in other nematode intron sequences has been described, both for *Haemonchus contortus* β-tubulin (Beech, Prichard & Scott, 1994) and for a number of *Ascaris* genes (Anderson & Jaenike, 1997). These findings were based on restriction site polymorphisms rather than primary sequence, and so cannot at this stage be directly compared to our observations on filarial intron variation.

Microfilarial sheath proteins: SHP-1 and SHP-5

Because morphological and behavioural variation appears most prominently in the microfilarial stage, Mf proteins from *B. malayi* are of particular interest with respect to their variability. The sheath of microfilariae is formed from the vestiges of the eggshell, and is found in some genera (*Brugia*, *Loa*, *Litomosoides*, *Wuchereria*) but not others (*Onchocerca*, *Acanthocheilonema*, *Dirofilaria*, *Mansonella*). In sheathed Mf, this structure represents the physical interface between host and parasite, and is therefore likely to be subject to immune pressure. This hypothesis can be tested by investigating whether sheath proteins shows higher sequence diversity than other filarial products.

We have recently been studying the SHP-1 antigen, originally named MF-22 after its molecular weight (Selkirk *et al.* 1991). Comparison of full-length sequences from *B. pahangi* (Selkirk *et al.* 1991) and *B. malayi* (Zahner *et al.* 1995) show extensive coding changes, including one-codon insertions/deletions (indels) in the repeat region of the protein. The majority of nucleotide substitutions are, in this case, non-synonymous. Overall, the two species show 10% amino acid sequence divergence (Table 3), the highest yet reported for filarial genes known to be orthologues. Moreover, the TRS strain EST dataset reveals that some copies of this gene from *B. malayi* have the *B. pahangi*-like indel pattern.

We have also examined the SHP-1 sequence by PCR amplification from genomic DNA of several isolates from Indonesia. These isolates have previously been characterized from the point of view of non-coding DNA markers (Underwood *et al.* 2000) but our work is the first to study protein coding sequences. We have found not only that there is more extensive sequence variation in natural *B. malayi* populations, including additional indels (Fig. 2), but that there is a previously unknown gene which shares sufficient sequence identity with SHP-1 to be amplified with the same primers.

This novel gene has been named SHP-5. Remarkably, its 5′ and 3′ ends are very similar to SHP-1, but the central domain is very different and the repeat sequence shows little relationship. Most importantly, SHP-5 sequences from different isolates show variation in amino acids and contain indels (Fig. 2), which with the preliminary data currently to hand appears to be no less extensive than that observed among SHP-1 sequences.

Microfilarial chitinases

An additional microfilarial protein of importance is chitinase (Fuhrman, 1995), which is expressed as 2 distinct forms in *B. malayi* (p70 and p75), and 3 forms in *B. pahangi* (Fuhrman, Lee & Dalamagas, 1995). The chitinase proteins are easily surface-labelled (Maizels *et al.* 1983) and monoclonal antibody p70/p75 (antibody MF1) confers passive protection on recipient animals (Fuhrman *et al.* 1992). There is a substantial level of sequence heterogeneity in these proteins, although the existence of multiple genes has so far prevented assignation of alleles and splice variants to any one locus. Thus, RT-PCR from *B. malayi* cDNA revealed two forms differing by 48-nt encoding a serine/threonine-rich repeat motif. Similar amplification from *B. pahangi* yielded a 42-nt (14aa)

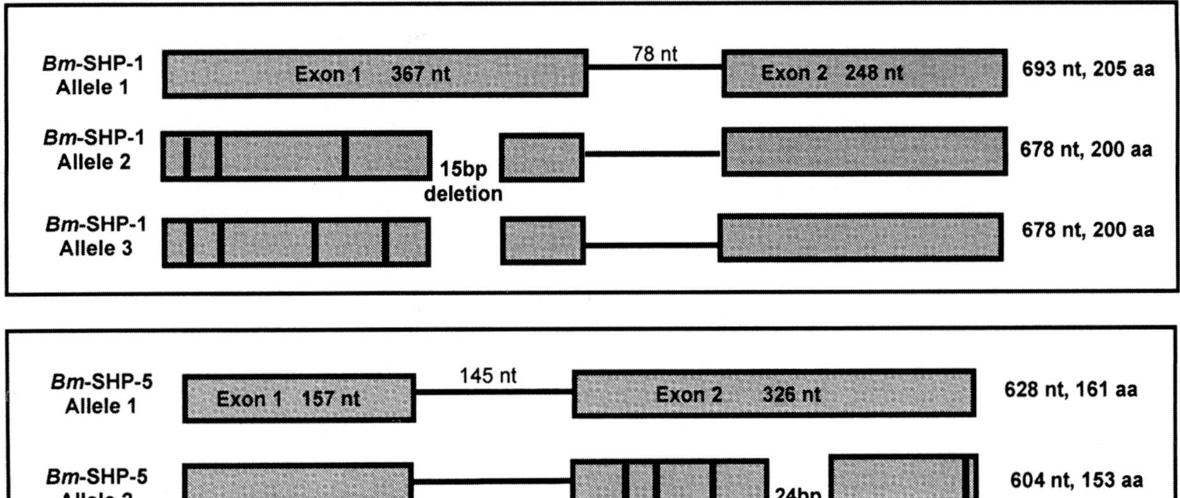

Fig. 2. Polymorphism of microfilarial sheath protein genes SHP-1 and SHP-5 from *Brugia malayi*. Allelic forms of two sheath protein genes, SHP-1 (also known as MF-22) and SHP-5 (also termed Shp-1a by J. Hirzmann and H. Zahner, Univ. Giessen, personal communication). Boxes represent exons, thin lines are introns with nucleotide lengths given. Vertical bars denote coding changes in sequence; synonymous substitutions are not shown. Alleles shown are from the TRS laboratory strain and isolates from Indonesia (Kurniawan-Atmadja *et al.* unpublished). Not to scale.

difference for a similar sequence motif (Arnold *et al.* 1996). Analysis of the multiple *B. malayi* ESTs for chitinase show a relatively high level of variants represented, indicating that a more extensive study of this gene family would be well worthwhile.

DIVERSITY OF *ONCHOCERCA* PARASITES (RIVER BLINDNESS)

Although the focus of this review is on lymphatic filariae, it is important to include *Onchocerca volvulus*, another major filarial parasite the adults of which occupy a subcutaneous niche in humans. Microfilariae infest the skin, from where a blackfly vector uptakes parasites to continue transmission. Primarily found in Africa, two biological types have been described: a less malignant, non-blinding forest form, and a more pathogenic, blinding savanna biotype (Duke, 1980; McMahon *et al.* 1988). Latin American *O. volvulus* is thought to have been imported from Africa in recent centuries, although it displays distinct preferences for local *Simulium* species over the African vector (Romeo De Leon & Duke, 1966). In the Upper Orinoco region of Venezuela, it has been suggested that a distinct biotype exists, defined by microfilarial morphology, isozyme pattern, and a high level of blood microfilaraemia (Botto, Arango & Yarzábal, 1984). Perhaps this instance should remind us that only a small fraction of parasite biodiversity has been sampled, even for a geographically restricted species such as *O. volvulus*.

Most molecular studies have concentrated on comparisons of the two African biotypes of *O. volvulus*, as this distinction is important in disease control. Isoenzyme analyses revealed a number of polymorphic loci, but no alleles unique to either type. Allele frequencies differ between forest and savanna isolates, but this cannot be used to distinguish individual worms (Flockhart *et al.* 1986). At the molecular level, a DNA probe for a repeat sequence has been described which hybridises only to the forest form (Erttmann *et al.* 1987), although success depends on conditions which discriminate between different copy numbers of similar repeat sequences in the two strains (Harnett *et al.* 1989; Meredith *et al.* 1989).

In terms of coding sequence polymorphisms, Keddie looked at 4 antigens comparing savanna/blinding (Ghana and Mali) and forest/non-blinding (Côte d'Ivoire and Liberia) strains, namely calreticulin, protein disulphide isomerase, RAL-2 and aspartyl protease inhibitor (Ov-API-1 or Ov33-3). None had any coding differences (Table 1), and the rate of synonymous substitution varied from 0 to 2·4 per 1000 nucleotides (Keddie *et al.* 1999). These findings of only limited diversity have been used to argue that *O. volvulus* has emerged from a recent bottleneck (Unnasch & Williams, 2000). It would be interesting, therefore, to compare sequence diversity of the homologous genes in other species for which no such restriction is thought to have occurred.

DIVERSITY OR UNIFORMITY?

It has previously been argued (Maizels & Lawrence, 1991) that the success of filarial parasites may depend on their inducing a form of immunological tolerance in their host. Such a state may place selective pressure on parasites to conform in antigenic terms, for to diversify may take them outside the protective shelter of tolerance and lead to immune recognition and destruction. Early evidence for such a purifying selection was drawn from examples such as GPX, discussed above, and appears to be supported by studies on several other filarial proteins which, like GPX, are associated with the established adult stage.

New data now emerging, however, highlights the opposite scenario. Microfilarial sheath proteins reveal a high level of polymorphism, although the allelic variants have yet to be shown to have any immunological distinction. Antibody staining studies on the microfilarial surface provide evidence that this stage displays some form of antigenic variation, although here the structural targets have yet to be identified. It is conceivable that while the adult worms are driven to uniformity, the microfilarial stage diversifies because it is under a very different form of selective pressure. Closer definition of the patterns of variation may allow us to consider exactly what these selective pressures may be.

CONCLUSION

Parasitologists have, with some honourable exceptions, been tardy in studying phenotypic polymorphism in helminths. Now that tools are available for sophisticated analyses at the molecular level, we anticipate major advances in this area. Data so far available are both scanty and patchy, revealing a spectrum of variability from total conservation to surprising levels of allelism. The latter instances (such as *H. contortus* P-glycoprotein and the *B. malayi* sheath proteins) should be studied with greater intensity if we are to probe the true extent of helminth genetic variation. More thought should be devoted to scanning the set of parasite-expressed proteins for those showing the highest level of diversity, so that variation is not sought only in those proteins which appear on our current understanding to be most likely candidates.

Once substantial datasets are in place, we may be in a position to address the key questions of what selective forces may be driving polymorphism, and what are the relative selective pressures exerted by host and vector (Read & Viney, 1996; Wakelin & Goyal, 1996; Anderson *et al.* 1998). Experimental genetic systems such as transgenesis for helminths are in their infancy, but if developed may allow variant forms of antigens to be functionally compared. Sophisticated manipulation of the host immune system is already possible, so that one can envisage at a future point being able to test not only whether particular variants are advantageous in immune evasion, but also which arm of the immune system they may have evolved to combat. The study of helminth polymorphisms on this broader stage, across the whole species in the wild, and driven by many possible forces from host, vector and environment, is sure to provide many such fascinating and insightful advances and make an essential contribution to the control and elimination of helminth diseases.

ACKNOWLEDGEMENTS

The authors thank the Wellcome Trust for support through a Programme Grant (RMM) and an International Research Development Award (AKA), and the European Commission (contract ICA4-2000-10195). We also thank Natalia Gomez-Escobar and Bill Gregory for permission to quote unpublished work on *B. malayi* genes.

REFERENCES

ANDERSON, T. J. C., BLOUIN, M. S. & BEECH, R. N. (1998). Population biology of parasitic nematodes: applications of genetic markers. *Advances in Parasitology* **41**, 219–283.

ANDERSON, T. J. C. & JAENIKE, J. (1997). Host specificity, evolutionary relationships and macrogeographic differentiation among *Ascaris* populations from humans and pigs. *Parasitology* **115**, 325–342.

ANDERSON, T. J. C., ROMERO-ABAL, M. E. & JAENIKE, J. (1993). Genetic structure and epidemiology of *Ascaris* populations: patterns of host affiliation in Guatemala. *Parasitology* **107**, 319–334.

ANDERSON, T. J. C., ROMERO-ABAL, M. E. & JAENIKE, J. (1995). Mitochondrial DNA and *Ascaris* microepidemiology: the composition of parasite populations from individual hosts, families and villages. *Parasitology* **110**, 221–229.

ARNOLD, K., VENEGAS, A., HOUSEWEART, C. & FUHRMAN, J. A. (1996). Discrete transcripts encode multiple chitinase isoforms in Brugian microfilariae. *Molecular and Biochemical Parasitology* **80**, 149–158.

BAIN, O., CHANDRASEKHARAN, S. A., PARTONO, F., MAK, J. W., ZHENG, H. J., SEO, B. S. & WU, S. H. (1989). Discrimination de souches géographiques de *Brugia malayi* périodique par l'ornementation cuticulaire des males. *Annales de Parasitologie Humaine et Comparée* **63**, 209–223.

BEECH, R. N., PRICHARD, R. K. & SCOTT, M. E. (1994). Genetic variability of the beta-tubulin genes in benzimidazole-susceptible and -resistant strains of *Haemonchus contortus*. *Genetics* **138**, 103–110.

BELLABY, T., ROBINSON, K. & WAKELIN, D. (1996). Induction of differential T-helper-cell responses in mice infected with variants of the parasitic nematode *Trichuris muris*. *Infection and Immunity* **64**, 791–795.

BELLABY, T., ROBINSON, K., WAKELIN, D. & BEHNKE, J. M. (1995). Isolates of *Trichuris muris* vary in their ability to elicit protective immune responses in mice. *Parasitology* **111**, 353–357.

BIANCO, A. E., ROBERTSON, B. D., KUO, Y.-M., TOWNSON, S. & HAM, P. (1990). Developmentally regulated expression and secretion of a polymorphic antigen by *Onchocerca* infective-stage larvae. *Molecular and Biochemical Parasitology* **39**, 203–212.

BIANCO, A. E., WU, Y. & JENKINS, R. E. (1995). *Onchocerca* spp: a "family" of secreted acidic proteins expressed by infective larvae in blackflies. *Experimental Parasitology* **81**, 344–354.

BLACKHALL, W. J., LIU, H. Y., XU, M., PRICHARD, R. K. & BEECH, R. N. (1998). Selection at a P-glycoprotein gene in ivermectin- and moxidectin-selected strains of *Haemonchus contortus*. *Molecular and Biochemical Parasitology* **95**, 193–201.

BLAXTER, M. L., ASLETT, M., GUILIANO, D., DAUB, J. & THE FILARIAL GENOME PROJECT (1999). Parasitic helminth genomics. *Parasitology* **118**, S39–S51.

BOLAS-FERNANDEZ, F. & WAKELIN, D. (1990). Infectivity, antigenicity and host responses to isolates of the genus *Trichinella*. *Parasitology* **100**, 491–497.

BOTTO, C., ARANGO, M. & YARZÁBAL, L. (1984). Onchocerciasis in Venezuela: prevalence of microfilaraemia in Amerindians and morphological characteristics of the microfilariae from the Upper Orinoco focus. *Tropenmedizin und Parasitologie* **35**, 167–173.

BUCKLEY, J. J. C. (1960). On *Brugia* gen. nov. for *Wuchereria* spp. of the malayi group i.e. *Wuchereria malayi* (Brug, 1927) *Wuchereria pahangi* Buckley and Edeson 1956 and *Wuchereria patei* Buckley, Nelson, Heisch 1958. *Annals of Tropical Medicine and Parasitology* **54**, 75–77.

COOKSON, E., BLAXTER, M. L. & SELKIRK, M. E. (1992). Identification of the major soluble cuticular protein of lymphatic filarial nematode parasites (gp29) as a secretory homolog of glutathione peroxidase. *Proceedings of the National Academy of Sciences, USA* **89**, 5837–5841.

COOKSON, E., TANG, L. & SELKIRK, M. E. (1993). Conservation of primary sequence of gp29, the major soluble cuticular glycoprotein, in three species of lymphatic filariae. *Molecular and Biochemical Parasitology* **58**, 155–160.

CURTIS, J. & MINCHELLA, D. J. (2000). Schistosome population genetic structure: when clumping worms is not just splitting hairs. *Parasitology Today* **16**, 68–71.

DUKE, B. O. L. (1980). Observations on *Onchocerca volvulus* in experimentally infected chimpanzees. *Tropenmedizin und Parasitologie* **31**, 41–54.

EDESON, J. F. B. & WHARTON, R. H. (1958). The experimental transmission of *Wuchereria malayi* from man to various animals on Malaya. *Transactions of the Royal Society of Tropical Medicine and Hygiene* **52**, 25–45.

ELARD, L., COMES, A. M. & HUMBERT, J. F. (1996). Sequences of β-tubulin cDNA from benzimidazole-susceptible and -resistant strains of *Teladorsagia circumcincta*, a nematode parasite of small ruminants. *Molecular and Biochemical Parasitology* **79**, 249–253.

ERTTMANN, K. D., UNNASCH, T. R., GREENE, B. M., ALBIEZ, E. J., BOATENG, J., DENKE, A. M., FERRARONI, J. J., KARAM, M., SCHULZ-KEY, H. & WILLIAMS, P. N. (1987). A DNA sequence specific for forest form *Onchocerca volvulus*. *Nature* **327**, 415–417.

FLOCKHART, H. A., CIBULSKIS, R. E., KARAM, M. & ALBIEZ, E. J. (1986). *Onchocerca volvulus*: enzyme polymorphism in relation to the differentiation of forest and savannah strains of this parasite. *Transactions of the Royal Society of Tropical Medicine and Hygiene* **80**, 285–292.

FRASER, E. M. & KENNEDY, M. W. (1991). Heterogeneity in the expression of surface-exposed epitopes among larvae of *Ascaris lumbricoides*. *Parasite Immunology* **13**, 219–225.

FUHRMAN, J. A. (1995). Filarial chitinases. *Parasitology Today* **11**, 259–261.

FUHRMAN, J. A., LANE, W. S., SMITH, R. F., PIESSENS, W. F. & PERLER, F. B. (1992). Transmission-blocking antibodies recognize microfilarial chitinase in brugian lymphatic filariasis. *Proceedings of the National Academy of Sciences, USA* **89**, 1548–1552.

FUHRMAN, J. A., LEE, J. & DALAMAGAS, D. (1995). Structure and function of a family of chitinase isozymes from Brugian microfilariae. *Experimental Parasitology* **80**, 672–680.

GILLEARD, J. S., DUNCAN, J. L. & TAIT, A. (1995). An immunodominant antigen on the *Dictyocaulus viviparus* L3 sheath surface coat and a related molecule in other strongylid nematodes. *Parasitology* **111**, 193–200.

GOYAL, P. K. & WAKELIN, D. (1993). Vaccination against *Trichinella spiralis* in mice using antigens from different isolates. *Parasitology* **107**, 311–317.

GREGORY, W. F., ATMADJA, A. K., ALLEN, J. E. & MAIZELS, R. M. (2000). The abundant larval transcript 1/2 genes of *Brugia malayi* encode stage-specific candidate vaccine antigens for filariasis. *Infection and Immunity* **68**, 4174–4179.

HACKETT, F., SIMPSON, A. J. G., OMER-ALI, P. & SMITHERS, S. R. (1987). Surface antigens of and cross-protection between two geographical isolates of *Schistosoma mansoni*. *Parasitology* **94**, 301–312.

HARNETT, W., CHAMBERS, A. E., RENZ, A. & PARKHOUSE, R. M. E. (1989). An oligonucleotide probe specific for *Onchocerca volvulus*. *Molecular and Biochemical Parasitology* **35**, 119–125.

HAWDON, J. M., JONES, B. F., HOFFMAN, D. R. & HOTEZ, P. J. (1996). Cloning and characterization of *Ancylostoma*-secreted protein. A novel protein associated with the transition to parasitism by infective hookworm larvae. *Journal of Biological Chemistry* **271**, 6672–6678.

HAWKING, F. (1975). Circadian and other rhythms of parasites. *Advances in Parasitology* **13**, 123–182.

HIRZMANN, J., SCHNAUFER, A., HINTZ, M., CONRATHS, F., STIRM, S., ZAHNER, H. & HOBOM, G. (1995). *Brugia* spp. and *Litomosoides carinii*: identification of a covalently cross-linked microfilarial sheath matrix protein (shp2). *Molecular and Biochemical Parasitology* **70**, 95–106.

HOEKSTRA, R., OTSEN, M., TIBBEN, J., LENSTRA, J. A. & ROOS, M. H. (2000). Transposon associated markers for the parasitic nematode *Haemonchus contortus*. *Molecular and Biochemical Parasitology* **105**, 127–135.

JOHNSTON, D. A., BLAXTER, M. L., DEGRAVE, W. M., FOSTER, J., IVENS, A. C. & MELVILL, S. E. (1999). Genomics and the biology of parasites. *BioEssays* **21**, 131–147.

JOSEPH, G. T., HUIMA, T. & LUSTIGMAN, S. (1998). Characterization of an *Onchocerca volvulus* L3-specific larval antigen, Ov-ALT-1. *Molecular and Biochemical Parasitology* **96**, 177–183.

KEDDIE, E. M., HIGAZI, T., BOAKYE, D., MERRIWEATHER, A., WOOTEN, M. C. & UNNASCH, T. R. (1999). *Onchocerca volvulus*: limited heterogeneity in the nuclear and mitochondrial genomes. *Experimental Parasitology* **93**, 198–206.

KWA, M. S. G., VEENSTRA, J. G. & ROOS, M. H. (1994). Benzimidazole resistance in *Haemonchus contortus* is correlated with a conserved mutation at amino acid 200 in β-tubulin isotype 1. *Molecular and Biochemical Parasitology* **63**, 299–303.

LAURIE, C. C. & STAM, L. F. (1994). The effect of an intronic polymorphism on alcohol dehydrogenase expression in *Drosophila melanogaster*. *Genetics* **138**, 379–385.

LESLIE, J. F., CAIN, G. D., MEFFE, G. K. & VRIJENHOEK, R. C. (1982). Enzyme polymorphism in *Ascaris suum* (Nematoda). *Journal of Parasitology* **68**, 576–587.

LOVERDE, P. T., DEWALD, J., MINCHELLA, D. J., BOSSHARDT, S. C. & DAMIAN, R. T. (1985). Evidence for host-induced selection in *Schistosoma mansoni*. *Journal of Parasitology* **71**, 297–301.

MACKENZIE, A. & QUINN, J. (1999). A serotonin transporter gene intron 2 polymorphic region, correlated with affective disorders, has allele-dependent differential enhancer-like properties in the mouse embryo. *Proceedings of the National Academy of Sciences, USA* **96**, 15251–15255.

MAIZELS, R. M. & LAWRENCE, R. A. (1991). Immunological tolerance: the key feature in human filariasis? *Parasitology Today* **7**, 271–276.

MAIZELS, R. M., BLAXTER, M. L. & SCOTT, A. L. (2001). Immunogenomics of filariasis: genes implicated in immune evasion and protective immunity. *Parasite Immunology* **23**, 327–344.

MAIZELS, R. M., GOMEZ-ESCOBAR, N., GREGORY, W. F., MURRAY, J. & ZANG, X. (2001). Immune evasion genes from filarial nematodes. *International Journal for Parasitology* **31**, 889–898.

MAIZELS, R. M., GREGORY, W. F., KWAN-LIM, G.-E. & SELKIRK, M. E. (1989). Filarial surface antigens: the major 29,000 mol.wt. glycoprotein and a novel 17,000–200,000 mol.wt. complex from adult *Brugia malayi* parasites. *Molecular and Biochemical Parasitology* **32**, 213–227.

MAIZELS, R. M., PARTONO, F., OEMIJATI, S., DENHAM, D. A. & OGILVIE, B. M. (1983). Cross-reactive surface antigens on three stages of *Brugia malayi*, *B. pahangi* and *B. timori*. *Parasitology* **87**, 249–263.

MCGREEVY, P. B., RATIWAYANTO, S., TUTI, S., MCGREEVY, M. M. & DENNIS, D. T. (1980). *Brugia malayi*: relationship between anti-sheath antibodies and amicrofilaremia in natives living in an endemic area of South Kalimantan, Borneo. *American Journal of Tropical Medicine and Hygiene* **29**, 553–562.

MCMAHON, J. E., SOWA, S. I., MAUDE, G. H. & KIRKWOOD, B. R. (1988). Onchocerciasis in Sierra Leone 2: a comparison of forest and savanna villages. *Transactions of the Royal Society of Tropical Medicine and Hygiene* **82**, 595–600.

MCMANUS, D. P. & BOWLES, J. (1996). Molecular genetic approaches to parasite identification: their value in diagnostic parasitology and systematics. *International Journal for Parasitology* **26**, 687–704.

MEREDITH, S. E. O., UNNASCH, T. R., KARAM, M., PIESSENS, W. F. & WIRTH, D. F. (1989). Cloning and characterization of an *Onchocerca volvulus* specific DNA sequence. *Molecular and Biochemical Parasitology* **36**, 1–10.

MOLONEY, N. A., GARCIA, E. G. & WEBBE, G. (1985). The strain specificity of vaccination with ultra violet attenuated cercariae of the Chinese strain of *Schistosoma japonicum*. *Transactions of the Royal Society of Tropical Medicine and Hygiene* **79**, 245–247.

MOLONEY, N. A., HINCHCLIFFE, P. & WEBBE, G. (1989). Cross protection between a laboratory passaged Chinese strain of *Schistosoma japonicum* and field isolates of *S. japonicum* from China. *Transactions of the Royal Society of Tropical Medicine and Hygiene* **83**, 83–85.

MURRAY, J., GREGORY, W. F., GOMEZ-ESCOBAR, N., ATMADJA, A. K. & MAIZELS, R. M. (2001). Expression and immune recognition of *Brugia malayi* VAL-1, a homologue of vespid venom allergens and *Ancylostoma* secreted proteins. *Molecular and Biochemical Parasitology* **118**, 89–96.

NADLER, S. A. (1986). Biochemical polymorphism in *Parascaris equorum*, *Toxocara canis* and *Toxocara cati*. *Molecular and Biochemical Parasitology* **18**, 45–54.

NADLER, S. A. (1990). Molecular approaches to studying helminth population genetics and phylogeny. *International Journal for Parasitology* **20**, 11–29.

NADLER, S. A. (1995). Microevolution and the genetic structure of parasite populations. *Journal of Parasitology* **81**, 395–403.

PALMIERI, J. R., PURNOMO, DENNIS, D. T. & MARWOTO, H. A. (1980). Filarid parasites of South Kalimantan (Borneo) Indonesia. *Wuchereria kalimantani* sp. n. (Nematoda: Filarioidea) from the silvered leaf monkey, *Presbytis cristatus* Eschscholtz 1921. *Journal of Parasitology* **66**, 645–651

PARTONO, F. (1987). The spectrum of disease in lymphatic filariasis. In *Filariasis* (ed. Everard, D. & Clark, S.), pp. 15–31. Chichester, Chichester.

PARTONO, F. & PURNOMO (1987). Periodicity studies of *Brugia malayi* in Indonesia: recent findings and a modified classification of the parasite. *Transactions of the Royal Society of Tropical Medicine and Hygiene* **81**, 657–662.

PRICHARD, R. (2001). Genetic variability following selection of *Haemonchus contortus* with anthelmintics. *Trends in Parasitology* **17**, 445–453.

QIANG, S., BIN, Z., SHU-HUA, X., ZHENG, F., HOTEZ, P. & HAWDON, J. M. (2000). Variation between ASP-1 molecules from *Ancylostoma caninum* in China and the United States. *Journal of Parasitology* **86**, 181–185.

RAVINDRAN, B., SATAPATHY, A. K. & SAHOO, P. K. (1994). Bancroftian filariasis – differential reactivity of anti-sheath antibodies in microfilariae carriers. *Parasite Immunology* **16**, 321–323.

READ, A. F. & VINEY, M. E. (1996). Helminth immunogenetics: why bother? *Parasitology Today* **12**, 337–343.

ROMEO DE LEON, J. & DUKE, B. O. (1966). Experimental studies on the transmission of Guatemalan and West African strains of *Onchocerca volvulus* by *Simulium ochraceum*, *S. metallicum* and *S. callidum*. *Transactions of the Royal Society of Tropical Medicine and Hygiene* **60**, 735–752.

SANGSTER, N. (1996). Pharmacology of anthelmintic resistance. *Parasitology* **113**, S201–S216.

SASA, M. (1976). *Human Filariasis. A Global Survey of Epidemiology and Control*. Baltimore, University Park Press.

SELKIRK, M. E., YAZDANBAKHSH, M., FREEDMAN, D., BLAXTER, M. L., COOKSON, E., JENKINS, R. E. & WILLIAMS, S. A. (1991). A proline-rich structural protein of the surface sheath of larval *Brugia filarial* nematode parasites. *Journal of Biological Chemistry* **266**, 11002–11008.

SEN, H. G. (1972). *Necator americanus*: behaviour in hamsters. *Experimental Parasitology* **32**, 26–32.

SHIMOGIRI, T., KONO, M., MANNEN, H., MIZUTANI, M. & TSUJI, S. (1998). Chicken ornithine transcarbamylase gene, structure, regulation, and chromosomal assignment: repetitive sequence motif in intron 3 regulates this enzyme activity. *Journal of Biochemistry (Tokyo)* **124**, 962–971.

SOLOMON, M. S. & HALEY, A. J. (1966). Biology of the rat nematode *Nippostrongylus brasiliensis* (Travassos, 1914). V. Characteristics of *N. brasiliensis* after serial passage in the laboratory mouse. *Journal of Parasitology* **52**, 237–241.

STAM, L. F. & LAURIE, C. C. (1996). Molecular dissection of a major gene effect on a quantitative trait: the level of alcohol dehydrogenase expression in *Drosophila melanogaster*. *Genetics* **144**, 1559–1564.

SU, Z. & DOBSON, C. (1997). Genetic and immunological adaptation of *Heligmosomoides polygyrus* in mice. *International Journal for Parasitology* **27**, 653–663.

TANG, L., SMITH, V. P., GOUNARIS, K. & SELKIRK, M. E. (1996). *Brugia pahangi*: the cuticular glutathione peroxidase (gp29) protects heterologous membranes from lipid peroxidation. *Experimental Parasitology* **82**, 329–332.

THE FILARIAL GENOME PROJECT (1999). Deep within the filarial genome: an update on progress in the Filarial Genome Project. *Parasitology Today* **15**, 219–224.

UNDERWOOD, A. P., SUPALI, T., WU, Y. & BIANCO, A. E. (2000). Two microsatellie loci from *Brugia malayi* show polymorphisms among isolates from Indonesia and Malaysia. *Molecular and Biochemical Parasitology* **106**, 299–302.

UNNASCH, T. R. & WILLIAMS, S. A. (2000). The genomes of *Onchocerca volvulus*. *International Journal for Parasitology* **30**, 543–552.

WAKELIN, D. & GOYAL, P. K. (1996). *Trichinella* isolates: parasite variability and host responses. *International Journal for Parasitology* **26**, 471–481.

WESCOTT, R. B. & TODD, A. C. (1966). Adaptation of *Nippostrongylus brasiliensis* to the mouse. *Journal of Parasitology* **52**, 233–236.

WILSON, T., EDESON, J. F. B., WHARTON, R. H., REID, J. A., TURNER, L. H. & LAING, A. B. G. (1959). The occurrence of two forms of *Wuchereria malayi* in man. *Transactions of the Royal Society of Tropical Medicine and Hygiene* **53**, 480–481.

ZAHNER, H., HOBOM, G. & STIRM, S. (1995). The microfilarial sheath and its proteins. *Parasitology Today* **11**, 116–120.

ZENG, W. & DONELSON, J. E. (1992). The actin genes of *Onchocerca volvulus*. *Molecular and Biochemical Parasitology* **55**, 207–216.

Variation and immunity to intestinal worms

D. WAKELIN*, S. E. FARIAS[1] *and* J. E. BRADLEY

[1] *School of Life and Environmental Sciences, University of Nottingham, Nottingham NG7 2RD, England. Department of Physiology and Biotechnology Centre, Federal University of Rio Grande do Sul, Brazil.*

SUMMARY

Genetically determined variation in host capacity to express resistance to a given parasite plays a major role in determining the outcome of infection. It can be assumed that the same is true of variation in parasites, but very much less is known of its influence on the host–parasite relationship. Phenotypic and genotypic variation within species of intestinal worms is now well documented, detailed studies having been made of parasites such as *Ascaris* in humans and trichostrongyles in domestic animals. However, the extent to which this variation affects the course of infection or the host immune response in these hosts is limited. Of the nematodes used as experimental models in laboratory rodents, detailed data on phenotypic or genotypic variation are limited to *Strongyloides* and *Trichinella*. Parasite variation is known to be subject to host-mediated selection, the emergence of anthelmintic resistance being a good example. Repeated passage has been used to select lines of parasite that survive in abnormal hosts or which show adaptation to host immunity. Experimental studies with *Trichinella* genotypes in mice have demonstrated the extent to which parasite variation influences the nature and degree of the host's immune and inflammatory responses, the complex interplay between immunogenicity and pathogenicity influencing both partners in the relationship. Recent studies with isolates of *Trichuris muris* have shown how parasite variation influences the capacity of mice to express the T helper cell responses necessary for resistance. Molecular differences between *T. muris* isolates have been shown in their excreted/secreted products as well as at the level of their DNA. Knowledge of the functional consequences of parasite variation will add to our understanding of host-parasite evolution as well as providing a rational basis for predicting the outcome of controls strategies that rest on the improvement of host resistance through vaccination or selective breeding.

Key words: Parasite variation, host immunity, selection, *Trichinella*, *Trichuris muris*.

INTRODUCTION

The outcome of interactions between particular hosts and particular parasites cannot be predicted simply from knowing the species involved. A wide variety of both exogenous and endogenous factors influences the balance of host–parasite relationships and determines the degree to which the fitness of one partner in the relationship is maintained at the expense of the other. At one extreme hosts may regulate or eliminate the parasite, at the other parasites may cause severe pathology or kill the host. All endogenous influences on host–parasite relationships have a genetic component, for example those that arise from responses to altered environmental conditions, to changes in nutritional levels, to reproductive events or to concurrent infections. Particular attention has been focused on genetic factors that influence the capacity of the host to respond protectively to infection through innate and adaptive immune responses. The extensive literature on this subject illustrates the degree to which host variation is now accepted as a major determinant of the outcome of host–parasite relationships and reflects the ease with which host variation can be manipulated as a variable in experimental systems involving laboratory or domestic animals. A common corollary of experimental approaches, however, is the use of parasites that often have had a restricted origin and have been maintained as lines by routine passage, thus potentially showing limited variability. It is particularly the case with experimental studies involving helminths that the emphasis on the influence of host variation has not often been matched by a corresponding interest in the influence attributable to parasite variation. That this is an artificial situation is obvious when one considers the wide, almost global distribution of many species of worms. Such geographical distributions must be accompanied by a very large degree of genotypic and phenotypic variation within parasite populations, but we are still largely ignorant of the impact that such variation has on host protective responses to infection. However, our growing understanding of the nature of immune responses to intestinal worms and of the ways in which these responses are initiated and regulated by the molecular characteristics of the parasites concerned, provides a framework for considering the likely consequences of parasite variation. Knowledge of these consequences could have important theoretical and practical implications for the host's immune response to infection. If genotypic variation within populations is reflected in phenotypic variation in those molecules that elicit immunity (im-

* Corresponding author: Tel: +0115 951 3232. Fax: +0115 951 3252. E-mail: D.Wakelin@nottingham.ac.uk

Parasitology (2002), **125**, S39–S50. © 2002 Cambridge University Press
DOI: 10.1017/S0031182002001440 Printed in the United Kingdom

munogens) or those that reduce or suppress immunity (immunomodulators), then this is likely to impact on the generation of host immune responses and therefore on the outcome of the host-parasite relationship. If genotypic, and consequent phenotypic, variation in worms can be influenced by selection pressures, then there is the possibility that worms may be able to adapt to immunity, whether acquired naturally or by vaccination.

Here we briefly review the evidence for genetic variation within natural populations of intestinal nematodes, describe examples where genotypic and phenotypic characteristics have been altered under selection pressure, and then focus on experimental studies which have provided data on the ways in which the complex interplay between host and parasite variation influences host immune and inflammatory responses. Since individuals vary in the effectiveness or the severity of their immune responses to infection, host immunity can be broadly categorized as *weaker* or *stronger*. Equally, as parasites vary in their capacity to elicit or modulate host responses, they can be categorized as being more or less *immunogenic*. The interactions between these host and parasite categories is discussed in relation to data from work with two genera of intestinal nematodes *Trichinella* and *Trichuris*.

GENOTYPIC AND PHENOTYPIC VARIATION IN INTESTINAL NEMATODES

Genotypic variation within natural populations of intestinal nematode species has been most intensively studied in *Ascaris* spp. (reviewed Anderson, Blouin & Beech, 1998), in trichostrongyles of domestic ruminants (reviewed Gasser & Newton, 2000) and in *Trichinella* spp. (see e.g. Zarlenga *et al.* 1999) using a variety of sequencing and PCR-based techniques. This work, and a number of other studies, has identified very considerable degrees of genotypic variation even within comparatively small population samples. For example, in 265 *Ascaris* taken from humans and pigs in two Guatemalan villages, Anderson, Romero-Abal & Jaenike (1995) recovered 42 distinct mitochondrial genotypes. Parasites with the same genotype occurred more frequently within particular individuals than chance predicted, suggesting either that these infections arose from ingestion of clustered eggs passed by individual females or that particular worm genotypes were more successful in establishing mature infections. Hawdon *et al.* (2001) similarly found evidence of considerable genotypic diversity in *Necator americanus* recovered from individuals living in four villages in China.

The extent of genetic variation within human intestinal nematodes will be influenced by the degree to which the parasites of individual hosts represent isolated populations, and the degree to which individuals exchange parasites. Both of these will be affected by migration, movement and intermixing between human populations in endemic areas. The situation with nematodes of domestic animals may be more complex because of the more extensive mass movement of livestock. Work with *Ostertagia ostertagi* in cattle showed that more than 98% of nucleotide diversity was found within populations (Blouin *et al.* 1992), a pattern repeated for *Haemonchus contortus* and *Trichostrongylus circumcincta* in sheep, but not found in a trichostrongyle nematode from deer (Blouin *et al.* 1995). Grant & Whittington (1994), using RFLP analysis, found extensive genetic variation both between and within laboratory and field strains of *Trichostrongylus colubriformis*. Interestingly, the laboratory strain, which one might have predicted to be less diverse, proved to be as polymorphic as the field strain. Hoekstra *et al.* (1997), using a PCR-based microsatellite approach, similarly found extensive genetic diversity within populations of *Haemonchus contortus* taken from four geographical regions.

The genus *Trichinella* is one of the most widely distributed of all nematodes. Although members of the genus show a remarkable degree of morphological similarity there are good grounds for considering that they fall into ten distinct genotypes, seven of which have been given species status (Murrell *et al.* 2000). The different genotypes show considerable diversity in terms of host range and in their biological characteristics (Kapel, 2000). Variation within and between the genotypes has been measured by a variety of PCR techniques using both random and specific primers (from internally transcribed spacers, mitochondrial and ribosomal DNA, specific antigens and microsatellites). Variation has been recorded within isolates of particular genotypes (e.g *T. spiralis*, *T. pseudospiralis* and *T. nelsoni*) in several geographically distinct localities (Nagano *et al.* 1999; Wu *et al.* 1999; La Rosa & Pozio, 2000; La Rosa *et al.* 2001).

Extensive intra-specific genetic diversity has also been recorded, using a PCR-RFLP technique, in populations of *Strongyloides ratti* collected from the UK, the major diversity being found within subsamples of the total population (Fisher & Viney, 1998). Diversity in *Strongyloides* is also seen in phenotypic life history characteristics. Chehresa, Beech & Scott (1997) described considerable phenotypic diversity in lines of *Heligmosomoides polygyryrus* that had been isolated from a starting laboratory population. This variation was reflected in different rates of establishment, development and reproduction. These examples, and many others in the literature, demonstrate that populations of intestinal nematodes do show considerable intra-specific genotypic and phenotypic variation.

GENOTYPIC AND PHENOTYPIC RESPONSES TO SELECTION

Anthelmintic resistance

Although there has been a number of studies concerned with phenotypic responses to selection, detailed analysis of the genetic correlates of the selection process is limited to the phenomenon of anthelmintic resistance in trichostrongyle parasites of domestic ruminants, particularly *H. contortus* (Prichard, 2001). The intensive use of anthelmintics has resulted in widespread resistance, affecting all of the major compounds. This is a textbook example of an external factor selecting a rare gene because it confers significant survival benefits, thus increasing its frequency within the population. Mass movements of ruminants, and their associated worms, within and between countries have contributed to the geographical spread of resistance. The genetic change that confers resistance to benzimidazole-based drugs is a point mutation resulting in the replacement of phenylalanine by tryosine at position 200 in the β-tubulin isotype 1 gene (Grant & Mascord, 1996). This mutation appears to carry no, or only low, fitness costs to the worm and, as a result, once established in populations, the mutation persists. A number of studies have examined the possibility that drug-resistant strains may show additional phenotypic differences, particularly whether they are more or less immunogenic or pathogenic than drug-susceptible lines. Kelly *et al.* (1978) reported that benzimidazole-resistant *H. contortus* was more pathogenic in sheep than a drug-susceptible isolate, but contrasting findings were reported by MacLean & Holmes (1987) working with resistant and susceptible isolates of *T. colubriformis* in gerbils. Maingi, Scott & Pritchard (1990) found that parasitological and pathological parameters of infection with *H. contortus* were positively correlated with increasing levels of thiabendazole resistance. More recent and well-controlled studies in sheep with a drug-resistant and drug-susceptible isolates of *Teladorsagia circumcincta* showed no significant differences in faecal egg output (Barrett, Jackson & Huntley, 1998), although infections with the susceptible isolate became patent earlier. Following removal of the worms and a single challenge infection there were no differences in worm burden or numbers of mucosal mast cells between sheep exposed to the two isolates. Mallet & Hoste (1995) reported that a drug-resistant strain of *T. colubriformis* showed a lower fecundity in rabbits than a susceptible strain, but elicited greater mucosal inflammation and, interestingly, secreted greater quantities of acetylcholinesterase. However, the two strains not only differed in terms of resistance to thiabendazole but also came from different countries. Although it is therefore not possible unambiguously to correlate phenotypic differences affecting host responses with drug resistance, these data do show important levels of differences within the same species that impact on the host response to infection.

Host range

Clear phenotypic changes in responses to selection have been established by several workers when adapting nematodes to alternative host species. In the 1960s Haley and colleagues (Haley, 1966; Solomon & Haley, 1966) adapted *Nippostrongylus brasiliensis*, a natural parasite of the rat, to mice and to hamsters by repeated passage – i.e. selecting those worms able to survive and reproduce in the abnormal host. The nature of this adaptation is unknown, but, as survival and reproduction of *N. brasiliensis* is determined by the levels of host immunity it may well have involved altered immunogenicity or greater tolerance to immune effector mechanisms. The human hookworm *Necator americanus* has been successfully adapted to the golden hamster, again by repeated passage (Sen & Seth, 1967; Behnke, Paul & Rajasekariah, 1986).

Physiological characteristics

Although attempts to increase the levels of adaptation of *Strongyloides ratti* from rats to mice by repeated passage were unsuccessful (Gemmill, Viney & Read, 2000) this species has been used in a variety of other experimental approaches involving selection (reviewed Viney, 2001). Lines established from individual females differ markedly in their propensity to develop *via* the heterogonic or homogonic route. By using individual lines that show a mixture of both developmental routes it has been shown that selection can convert them into following primarily one or the other routes within a comparatively small number of generations. Switching between developmental routes is influenced by external temperature and by host immunity, and sensitivity to these triggers is again variable between lines. A similar interplay between temperature and immunity is known to affect the propensity of larval *Ostertagia ostertagi* to undergo arrested development in the mammalian host, although this may be a characteristic only of certain (temperate) isolates (Gibbs, 1986).

Response to host immunity

Other phenotypic changes that can clearly be related to host immunity as a selection pressure include the altered acetylcholinesterase isoenzyme pattern seen in *N. brasiliensis* worms as the rat host develops immunity during a primary infection (Edwards,

Burt & Ogilvie, 1971). The functional significance of this change is not known, but it has been shown that worms developing in immune rats (Ogilivie, 1972) or worms established through trickle, rather than single pulse, infections (Jenkins & Phillipson, 1972) become adapted to the immune host, elicit a reduced immune response and survive longer. This characteristic of reduced immunogenicity (and presumably that of altered acetylcholinesterase production) represents a phenotypic rather than a genotypic change as infections with the progeny of adapted worms are expelled by host immunity in the normal way.

Genotypic changes arising from adaptation to host immunity were reported by Dobson and colleagues, who carried out a long series of experiments to establish lines of *Heligmosomoides polygrus* (*Nematospiroides dubius*) by repeated passage through mice of different status (naïve, immune from single or challenge infections) as well as mice of different genotypes (Dobson & Owen, 1977). These selections resulted in lines of worms that showed a number of heritable phenotypic changes. Lines selected in the most immune mice showed better survival and reproduction in immune hosts (Dobson & Tang, 1991) and elicited lower antibody and inflammatory responses (Su & Dobson, 1997). The precise expression of these changes was quite strongly influenced by the genotype of the host, presumably mediated through variation in levels of genetically-determined resistance.

INTESTINAL NEMATODES AND IMMUNITY

Human hosts

Infections with intestinal nematodes stimulate strong immune responses in all hosts, but the relation of these responses to protection against infection remains unclear in all but a few cases. In general, infections appear to elicit weaker protective responses in humans than in other host groups, although whilst this may be true for populations it probably does not apply at the level of individuals (Maizels *et al.* 1993). It is true of all intestinal nematode infections that worms are distributed very unevenly within a population. Distributions are aggregated, which implies that certainly some individuals in populations living in endemic areas remain worm free, or sustain only small infections, despite frequent exposure to infection. This pattern of infection makes it difficult to draw conclusions about the possible influences of worm population variation on host immunity. However, there are data from work with *Ascaris* and *Trichuris* that suggest both that worm variation exists and that it may be important in terms of the host–parasite relationship. Fraser & Kennedy (1991) found variation in expression of surface antigens of *A. lumbricoides* infective larvae when these were exposed to antibody from the host population from which the larvae originated. Binding of antibody from an individual donor to surface antigens showed heterogeneity between larvae, suggesting either polymorphism in these antigens or differences in their expression. The antibodies concerned would have been elicited by the somatic rather than the intestinal stages of the worms, but the target antigens would presumably represent the repertoire determined by the worm's genome. It has been reported that adult *A. lumbricoides* from different geographical regions show striking differences in female worm fecundity (Hall & Holland, 2000). The mean worm burden in children from Bangladesh was 20·2 compared with 12·6 from Nigeria. However, the mean faecal egg counts were 2473 and 13609, respectively. It is tempting to implicate host immunity and differences in worm immunogenicity as casual factors, although there are no data to support this. Antigenic variation, detectable by immunoblotting with plasma from individual hosts, was found at the level of individual *T. trichiura* worms taken from the population present within the plasma donor (Currie *et al.* 1998).

Domestic ruminants

The greater control over experimental variables that is possible with the use of domestic livestock or experimental rodents makes it easier to devise experiments that look for evidence of parasite variation in the induction and expression of host immunity. Despite this, relatively few workers have exploited these approaches. The defined antigens developed as a vaccine candidate for *H. contortus* have been used in a comparative assay of the level of protection achieved in Australian lambs vaccinated with antigen (H11 – a gut membrane-derived molecule) prepared from British and Australian sources (Newton *et al.* 1995). Both antigen preparations protected well, but that from Australian worms gave rather better protection than antigen from British worms, protection from intra-muscular or subcutaneous administration being 75·5 and 87·7% (Australian), 60 and 55·9% (British). No major antigenic differences were detected by SDS-PAGE analysis.

Laboratory mice

The ability to *H. polygyrus* lines selected by passage through resistant mice to survive better in more resistant hosts could reflect reduced immunogenicity (as suggested for *N. brasiliensis* – see above), increased immunomodulation (it is known that *H. polygyrus* promotes its survival in this way – Behnke, Hannah & Pritchard, 1983; Telford *et al.*, 1998) or an enhanced ability to resist the harmful actions of effector mechanisms (*H. polygyrus* produces significant levels of antoxidants – Smith & Bryant, 1986). Tang, Dobson & McManus (1995) attempted to correlate phenotypic differences with molecular characteristics of worms selected by passage in a variety of mice, but although protein and antigen profiles showed differences between worms selected by passage through resistant as compared with naïve mice, no clear correlations were apparent between the profiles and worm phenotype.

The *H. polygyrus* used in almost all experimental work, derived initially from *Peromyscus maniculatus*, is one of four closely related sub-species and is correctly designated as *H. polygyrus bakeri*. Comparative studies using laboratory mice and the field mouse *A. sylvaticus* as hosts for this sub-species and *H. p. polygyrus* from *A. sylvaticus* revealed strongly contrasting patterns of parasite development and survival (Quinnell, Behnke & Keymer, 1991). *H. p. bakeri* survived well in laboratory mice but poorly in field mice, despite establishing well initially. In contrast *H. p. polygyrus*, survived in field mice but established very poorly in laboratory mice. Immunosuppressive treatment with corticosteroid allowed survival in all cases, suggesting that the failure of a given sub species to survive in the 'wrong' host was immune-mediated and therefore a reflection of differential immunogenicity compared with the native sub species.

VARIATION AND IMMUNITY IN *TRICHINELLA* INFECTIONS

The taxonomy of the genus *Trichinella* is based on both genotypic and phenotypic characteristics. Among the latter is the capacity to induce cyst formation in the muscles, which quite clearly delineates the majority of genotypes from *T. pseudospiralis* and *T. papuae*, neither of which forms cysts. Phenotypic characteristics relevant to the intestinal phase include its duration, the duration and level of female worm fecundity, the region of the intestine occupied by the worms and the degree of pathology associated with infection. All of these are known to be influenced by the host immune response and are therefore likely to be variable if there is variation within genotypes in the expression of antigens or immunomodulators.

There have been relatively few studies of immune responses to *Trichinella* genotypes in hosts other than laboratory mice. Differences in the antibody responses of pigs infected with Spanish origin *T. spiralis* and *T. britovi* were described by Bolas-Fernandez *et al.* (1993). Kapel & Gamble (2000) made a more detailed study in pigs infected with eight genotypes. *T. spiralis* was found to be the most infective genotype, giving a mean larval burden of 427 larvae/g body weight, *T. murrelli* and the genotype T6 being minimally infective producing a maximum burden of 5 larvae/g. The level and time course of antibody responses against ES antigens varied significantly between the genotypes, being, overall, highest against antigens from the homologous parasite. A similar study was made using nine genotypes in wild boars (Kapel, 2001) and again marked differences were found in antibody response, particularly during the post-intestinal phase of infection. A comparison of responses to nine genotypes carried out in rats by Malakauskas, Kapel & Webster (2000) showed that, although all became established, infectivity varied considerably. *T. spiralis* and three genotypes of *T. pseudospiralis* had the greatest infectivity, the others (*T. nativa*, *T. britovi*, *T. murrelli*, *T. nelsoni* and T6) showed low or negligible infectivity. The three genotypes of *T. pseudospiralis* showed differences in infectivity, particularly when this was measured in terms of larval survival over a 40-week period.

The ease with which *Trichinella* infections can be established in mice has resulted in a relatively large literature dealing with the influence of inter- and intra-genotypic variation on host responses (reviewed Wakelin & Goyal, 1996). Among more recent studies are those of Goyal & Wakelin (1993*a*, *b*) who described variations in infectivity and immunogenicity of different geographical isolates of *T. spiralis* when used to infect a single mouse strain. Although the isolates cross-immunized there were isolate-specific differences in the ability to elicit levels of immunity to challenge. In mice given single primary infections there were differences in levels of serum parasite-specific antibodies (IgG1, IgG2a, IgE) and inflammatory responses (mucosal mastocytosis, peripheral eosinophilia). In a subsequent paper, Goyal, Hermanek & Wakelin (1944) followed cytokine responses in mesenteric lymphocytes from infected mice and found that the isolates generating the greatest immune and inflammatory responses showed the earliest switch from a type 1 to a type 2 cytokine profile.

One of the most striking genotype-dependent differences in infectivity was observed when mice were infected with *T. spiralis* or *T. nativa* (a species found in wild animals in northern latitudes). *T. nativa* was expelled very rapidly from mice and reproduced poorly, but survival and reproduction were considerably improved when mice were immunesuppressed by corticosteroid treatment (Fig. 1) indicating that the genotypes differed in their immunogenicity. These two genotypes can be differentiated by SDS-PAGE and immunoblot analysis of larval homogenates, but no direct correlation with the greater immunogenicity in *T. nativa* has been established (Bolas-Fernandez & Wakelin, 1989). Differences in the IgG3 (anti-carbohydrate) res-

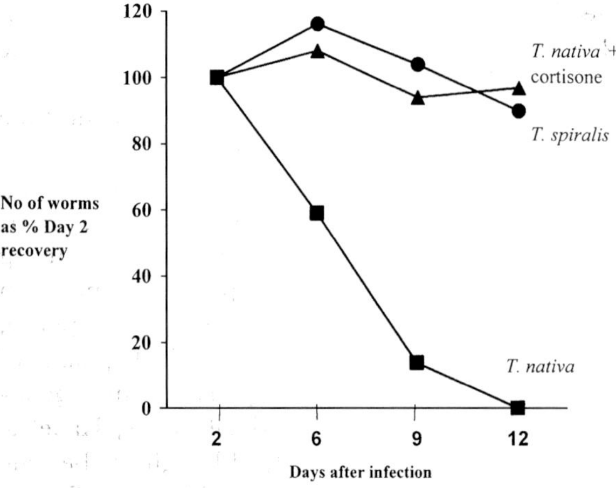

Fig. 1. Differential survival of *Trichinella* genotypes in NIH mice reflects differential immunogenicity. Two groups of mice were infected with 300 larvae of *T. spiralis* (●) or *T. nativa* (■). An additional group of *T. nativa*-infected mice was immunosuppressed with cortisone acetate (▲). Worm recoveries are shown as a percentage of the numbers present at day 2. (Data from Bolas-Fernandez & Wakelin, 1989).

ponses of mice infected with genotypes including *T. spiralis* and *T. nativa*, have been described by Dea-Ayueal *et al.* (2000).

Although there has been, and continues to be, some debate about species identity in the cyst-forming genotypes of *Trichinella*, the species status of *T. pseudospiralis* has been readily accepted because of the distinctive characteristics of its muscle phase. As with the other *Trichinella* species there is evidence of molecular and genetic diversity between isolates of *T. pseudospiralis* taken from different regions (Finland, France, Kazakhstan, Russia, Tasmania, USA – La Rosa *et al.* 2001). Differences have also been recorded in aspects of the host response to infection. *T. pseudospiralis* has a marked immunosuppressive influence on the host, and this down regulates inflammatory responses to both the intestinal and muscle phases of infection (Stewart, 1989). A comparison of inflammatory responses induced in mice by a long-established American and a recent Australian isolate showed that the latter induced less inflammation in the intestine but more in the muscle; both isolates produced considerably less inflammation than *T. spiralis* (Alford *et al.* 1998). When concurrent infections were established between *T. spiralis* and each isolate, muscle inflammation was reduced to a much greater degree by the American isolate. It is not clear whether the biological characteristics of the American isolate may reflect its long-term passage through mice (> 20 years), and the nature of the differences in anti-inflammatory capacity is not known. There is evidence that the immune suppression associated with infection of the American *T. pseudospiralis* reflects the induction of elevated plasma corticosterone levels (Stewart *et al.* 1988) and it is therefore possible that the two isolates differ in this property.

VARIATION AND IMMUNITY IN *TRICHURIS* INFECTIONS

Species of *Trichuris* occur in many mammalian hosts but, unlike *Trichinella*, show high host specificity. Apart from evidence for intraspecific antigen variation within the human *Trichuris* (*T. trichiura* – Currie *et al.* 1998) nothing is known about species other than *T. muris*, a natural parasite of murine hosts that has been widely used as an laboratory model.

Immunity to T. muris

T. muris elicits strong protective immune responses in the majority of laboratory mouse strains, and these result in the elimination of worms before they reach patency. Certain inbred strains, however (e.g. B10.BR, AKR) are permissive – i.e. they remain susceptible to infection and allow the worms to become sexually mature (Else & Wakelin, 1986). Recent work has shown that mouse strains that express resistance to *T. muris* infections characteristically develop immune responses mediated by T lymphocytes of the T helper 2 (Th2) subset, whereas permissive mice express responses mediated by Th1 cells (Grencis, 1996). The mechanisms underlying resistance are still undefined, but under the appropriate circumstances it can be shown that immunity is transferable with both T cells and antibodies separately (Else & Grencis, 1999; Blackwell & Else, 2001). Resistance and susceptibility are under strong genetic control, involving both MHC-linked and non-MHC (background) genes (Else & Wakelin, 1988). Some resistant mice expel worms early in infection (e.g. NIH mice within two weeks) others take one to two weeks longer (e.g. BALB/c and CBA). Expulsion of worms before week four of infection appears to be critical – mice unable to do this not only fail to expel a primary infection, but fail also to eliminate a subsequent challenge. Such permissive mice appear anergic to *T. muris* antigens (Soltys, Goyal & Wakelin, 1999), and there is evidence that the switch from resistance to permissiveness, and the corresponding alteration in cellular immunity, may be induced by factors released from the maturing worms (Grencis & Entwistle, 1997).

The stimulation of protective immunity requires exposure of the mouse to infections that are above a threshold level (approximately 10 eggs – Wakelin, 1973). Below this level worms survive to sexual maturity. There is a strong correlation between the level of infection experienced and the Th response elicited in the mouse, low level infection up-regulating Th1 responses, higher levels a Th2 response (Bancroft, Else & Grencis, 1994).

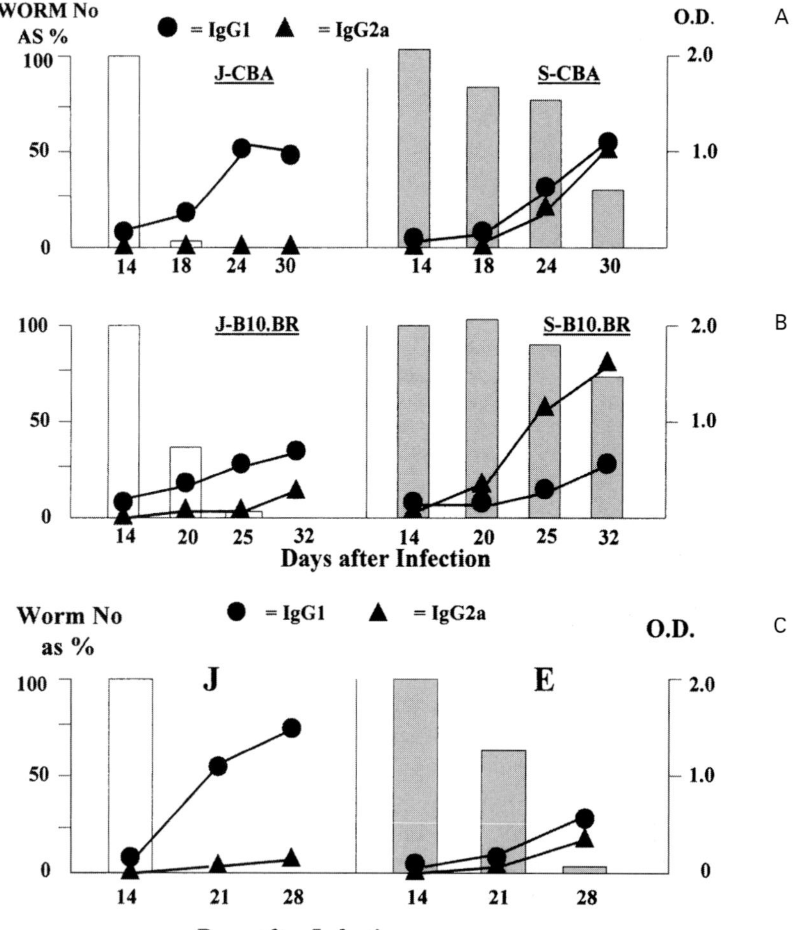

Fig. 2. Time course of infection (histograms) and IgG isotype responses (line graphs) of *Trichuris muris* isolates in mice of different genotypes. Worm numbers are given as a % of the day 14 recovery. ELISA values are given as optical density (O.D.). (Data from Bellaby *et al.* 1996). A,B. Resistant CBA and permissive B10.BR mice infected with the Japanese (J) or Sobreda (S) isolates. C. C57B/10 mice infected with the Japanese (J) or Edinburgh (E) isolates.

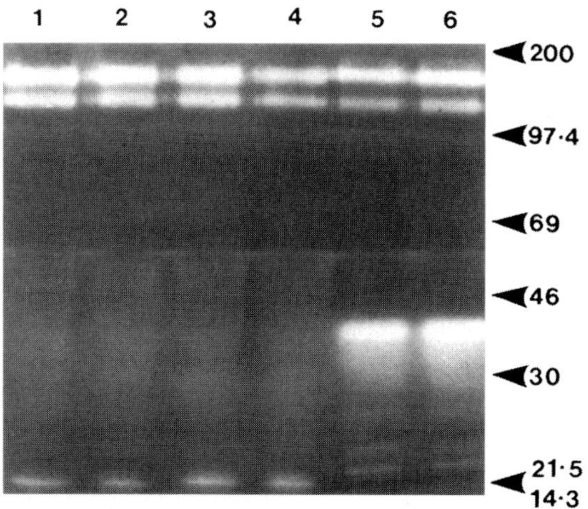

Fig. 3. Proteolytic activity of excretory/secretory material from the Edinburgh (lanes 1, 2) Japanese (lanes 3, 4), or Sobreda (lanes 5, 6) isolates of *Trichuris muris* run on a 12% SDS-polyacrylamide resolving gel containing 0·1% gelatin. After separation the proteins were renatured and incubated at 37 °C at pH 7·0 for 48 hours.

Behaviour of T. muris *isolates in laboratory mice*

The data summarized above have come from work with one particular laboratory-maintained isolate, obtained initially in 1954 from wild *Mus musculus* in Edinburgh Zoo (the E isolate) and maintained subsequently in immunesuppressed or immunodeficient laboratory mice. Two other isolates are also now available. The J isolate is derived from a batch of the E isolate sent in the 1960s to the USA and then, in 1971, made available to Y. Ito in Japan and passaged in immunosuppressed mice ever since. These isolates have therefore been maintained separately for some 60–100 generations. The third (S) isolate was recovered from *Mus spretus* in Portugal by J. M. Behnke in 1992 and has since been maintained in Nottingham in immunosuppressed mice.

The three isolates of *T. muris* show quite different patterns of infection in laboratory mouse strains and elicit different immune responses in the host (Bellaby *et al.* 1995; Bellaby, Robinson & Wakelin, 1996;

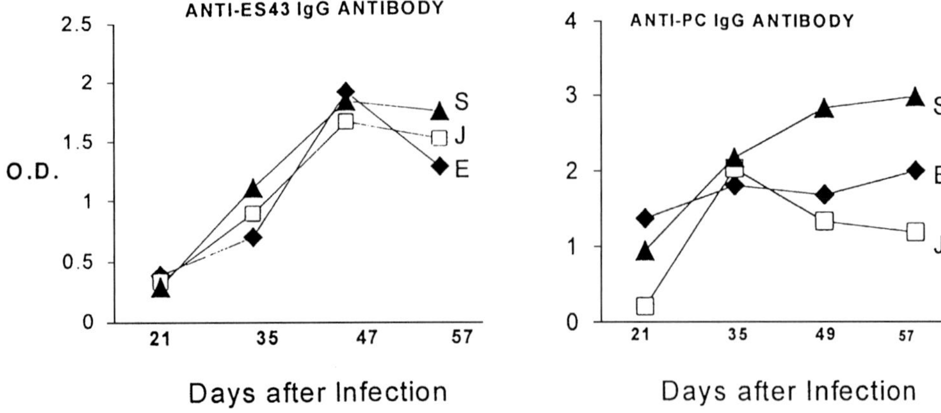

Fig. 4. IgG antibody responses of B10.BR mice infected with the Japanese (J), Edinburgh (E) or Sobreda (S) isolates of *Trichuris muris*. Sera were tested in ELISA against a purified preparation of the major immunogen from each isolate (43 kDa molecule from excretory/secretory (ES) material) and against a BSA-Phosphorylcholine (PC) conjugate. ELISA values are given in terms of optical density (O.D.).

Koyama & Ito, 1996, 2001). Key features of infections with the J and S isolates are illustrated in Fig. 2a. The J isolate is the most immunogenic of the three isolates and as a consequence is expelled most rapidly by mice that are genetically resistant, e.g. CBA. In these mice infection generates an IgG1 antibody response, a Th2-dependent isotype, with little or no IgG2a. J isolate worms are also expelled before patency in genetically permissive B10.BR, again with a predominantly IgG1 response. The S isolate appears to be the least immunogenic (or the most immunosuppressive), sexually mature infections developing even in genetically resistant mice. With this infection CBA mice develop similar IgG1 and IgG2a (Th1-dependent) responses. In B10.BR mice infections are chronic and the antibody response is dominated by IgG2a. The E isolate occupies a position that is intermediate between the other two, being expelled more slowly than J from resistant mice and surviving less well than S in permissive mice. The difference between the two isolates is clearly seen when they are used to infect C57BL/10 (B10) mice, which themselves are intermediate in resistance between CBA and B10.BR (Fig. 2b). The threshold level of infection necessary to elicit immunity differs between isolates. Thus with the J isolate, infections as low as 25 or 12·5 eggs trigger protective responses that result in the loss of worms from resistant CBA mice (mean recoveries day 35 were 0·45 and 0·73, respectively) in contrast similar infections with the S isolate result in the establishment of mature worm infections (mean recoveries 8·2 and 3·6).

These striking isolate-dependent differences in host–parasite relationship must reflect molecular differences associated with the induction or suppression of immune responses. Our laboratory at Nottingham has begun to look for evidence of such differences and current findings are summarized below.

Evidence of molecular differences between T. muris *isolates*

Small differences between isolates can be detected when worm homogenates and excretory-secretory material are analysed by SDS-PAGE. That some of these differences are functionally significant is supported by the fact that differences in antibody recognition are apparent when separated proteins from each isolate are blotted with homologous or heterologous sera from infected mice. In addition there are differences in patterns of serine protease activity when homogenate and ES material are run on substrate gels (Fig. 3). On SDS-PAGE all of the isolates show a major band at 43 kDA, a component known from previous studies to be an important immunogen. However, N-terminal sequencing of this component has failed to show any sequence difference between the isolates, suggesting the possibility that functionally important differences may exist in other molecules. A number of the components that separate on SDS-PAGE are glycosylated and some of these carry phosphorylcholine (PC), a molecule with potent immunomodulatory properties (Harnett *et al.* 1999). Resistant CBA and permissive B10.BR mice infected with each of the three isolates show very different patterns of anti-PC antibody responses, and in B10.BR these patterns differ strikingly between the isolates (Fig. 4), suggesting significant differences in PC presentation between them.

The Random Amplified Polymorphic DNA (RAPD) PCR technique has been used to look for genetic differences between the three isolates. A number of primers have revealed major band differences both with DNA from batches of small numbers (10) of worms and with DNA from individual worms (Fig. 5). These will provide markers for more detailed studies on the genetic basis of the phenotypic differences between the

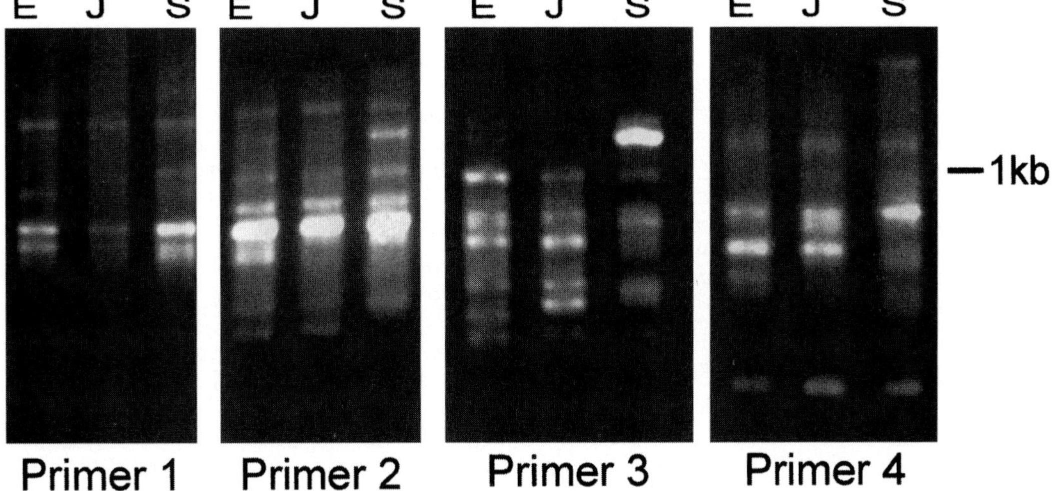

Fig. 5. Gel of RAPD-PCR products using four random primers and DNA from the Edinburgh (E), Japanese (J) and Sobreda (S) isolates of *Trichuris muris*. The results from each primer show major band differences between the isolates. The marker indicates MW in base pairs. Primer 1 – GACCGCTTGT; Primer 2 – CAGCACCCAC; Primer 3 – ACCCCCACAC; Primer 4 – GTCACGTCTC.

isolates. One approach will be to produce hybrids between the isolates and then monitor the segregation of phenotypic and genetic markers.

CONCLUSIONS

Intestinal nematodes, like all organisms, show considerable intraspecific genetic diversity. We now know that at least some of this diversity is reflected in phenotypic differences that affect the host–parasite relationship and that these differences can be subject to selection pressures originating from the host. The best studied example concerns the genetic and molecular basis of anthelmintic resistance in trichostrongyle nematodes, and this provides a model for the capacity of these parasites to respond to intense selection pressure. The evidence from this example is that nematodes can respond rapidly to selection, and this is confirmed by the data from work with the isolates of *T. muris* described above. In the absence of externally applied drug treatment the other major selection pressure acting on intestinal worms is the host's immune response. Although the evidence for protective immunity remains weak in humans, the evidence from experimental studies, and the principle of biological economy, suggest that host-protective responses act as a major environmental constraint on all intestinal nematodes. It can therefore by expected that there will be selection for those genotypes that survive and reproduce best in hosts of a given response phenotype. Selection may increase or decrease immunogenicity, or increase or decrease immunomodulatory ability, depending on which is most likely to optimize parasite fitness.

At present there are remarkably few data to provide a picture of the relationship between variation and immune responses as these relate to intestinal nematodes. The bulk of the data comes from experimental studies in mice with a handful of parasite species. Nevertheless these studies have provided a framework for future work that will have both theoretical and practical value. It is important, given the limitation on chemotherapeutic control, to quantify the ability of worm populations to modify their immunogenicity (or their immunmodulatory ability) from the standpoint of potential vaccine usage. Equally, it is important from the point of view of parasite population studies to understand how evolution acts on both host and parasite to optimize the fitness of each. This is not necessarily achieved by simply maximizing host resistance and minimizing parasite immunogenicity. All parasitism causes a loss of host resources. These arise from the costs of mounting immune and inflammatory responses, from the effects these may have on digestion, absorption and utilization of nutrients (a factor of major importance with intestinal infections) and from the loss of resources directly to the parasites themselves. Hosts must establish a trade-off between all of these factors to achieve maximum fitness in the face of continual exposure to infection. In turn, parasites must trade off the benefits of increased survival from reduced immunogenicity (or greater immunomodulation) against the possibility that the host may succumb to over infection. As seen very clearly with *Trichinella*, moderate immunogenicity may prevent over-infection (and keep out competing genotypes) but it carries the risk of eliciting immunopathological responses in the very environment that the parasites occupy. Knowledge of how specific genes in intestinal nematodes contribute to these crucial questions of host and parasite adaptation will lead to a much greater understanding of the population biology of this important group of parasites, as well as of the evolutionary pressures acting on their host–parasite relationships.

ACKNOWLEDGEMENT

Dr S. E. Farias is a recipient of a CAPES post-doctoral fellowship.

REFERENCES

ALFORD, K., OBENDORF, D. L., FREDEKING, T. M., HAEHLING, E. & STEWART, G. L. (1998). Comparison of the inflammatory responses of mice infected with American and Australian *Trichinella pseudospiralis* or *Trichinella spiralis*. *International Journal for Parasitology* **28**, 343–348.

ANDERSON, T. J., BLOUIN, M. S. & BEECH, R. N. (1998). Population biology of parasitic nematodes: applications of genetic markers. *Advances in Parasitology* **41**, 219–282.

ANDERSON, T. J., ROMERO-ABAL, M. E. & JAENIKE, J. (1995). Mitochondrial DNA and *Ascaris* microepidemiology: the composition of parasite populations from individual hosts, families and villages. *Parasitology* **110**, 221–229.

BANCROFT, A. J., ELSE, K. J. & GRENCIS, R. K. (1994). Low-level infection with *Trichuris muris* significantly affects the polarization of the CD4 response. *European Journal of Immunology* **2444**, 3113–3118.

BARRETT, F., JACKSON, F. & HUNTLEY, J. F. (1998). Pathogenicity and immunogenicity of different isolates of *Teladorsagia circumcincta*. *Veterinary Parasitology* **76**, 95–104.

BEHNKE, J. M., HANNAH, J. & PRITCHARD, D. I. (1983). *Nematospiroides dubius* in the mouse: evidence that adult worms depress the expression of homologous immunity. *Parasite Immunology* **5**, 397–408.

BEHNKE, J. M., PAUL, V. & RAJASEKARIAH, G. R. (1986). The growth and migration of *Necator americanus* following infection of neonatal hamsters. *Transactions of the Royal Society of Tropical Medicine and Hygiene* **80**, 146–149.

BELLABY, T., ROBINSON, K. & WAKELIN, D. (1996). Induction of differential T-helper-cell responses in mice infected with variants of the parasitic nematode *Trichuris muris*. *Infection and Immunity* **64**, 791–795.

BELLABY, T., ROBINSON, K., WAKELIN, D. & BEHNKE, J. M. (1995). Isolates of *Trichuris muris* vary in their ability to elicit protective immune responses to infection in mice. *Parasitology* **111**, 353–357.

BLACKWELL, N. M. & ELSE, K. J. (2001). B cells and antibodies are required for resistance to the parasitic gastrointestinal nematode parasite *Trichuris muris*. *Infection and Immunity* **69**, 3860–3868.

BLOUIN, M. S., DAME, J. B., TARRANT, C. A. & COURTNEY, C. H. (1992). Unusual population genetics of a parasitic nematode; mtDNA variation within and among populations. *Evolution* **46**, 470–476.

BLOUIN, M. S., YOWELL, C. A., COURTNEY, C. H. & DAME, J. B. (1995). Host movement and the genetic structure of populations of parasitic nematodes. *Genetics* **141**, 1007–1014.

BOLAS-FERNANDEZ, F. & WAKELIN, D. (1989). Infectivity of *Trichinella* isolates in mice is determined by host immune responsiveness. *Parasitology* **99**, 83–88.

BOLAS-FERNANDEZ, F., ALBARRAN-GOMEZ, E., NAVARRETE, I. & MARTINEZ-FERNANDEZ, A. R. (1993). Dynamics of porcine humoral responses to experimental infections by Spanish *Trichinella* isolates: comparison of three larval antigens in ELISA. *Journal of Veterinary Medicine Series B* **40**, 223–229.

CHEHRESA, A., BEECH, R. N. & SCOTT, M. E. (1997). Life-history variation among lines isolated from a laboratory population of *Heligmosomoides polygyrus bakeri*. *International Journal for Parasitology* **27**, 541–551.

CURRIE, R. M., NEEDHAM, C. S., DRAKE, L. J., COOPER, E. S. & BUNDY, D. A. (1998). Antigenic variability in *Trichuris trichiura* populations. *Parasitology* **117**, 347–353.

DEA-AYUELA, M. A., MARTINEZ-FERNANDEZ, A. R. & BOLAS-FERNANDEZ, F. (2000). Comparison of IgG3 responses to carbohydrates following mouse infection or immunization with six species of *Trichinella*. *Journal of Helminthology* **74**, 884–889.

DOBSON, C. & OWEN, M. E. (1977). Influence of serial passage on the infectivity and immunogenicity of *Nematospiroides dubius* in mice. *International Journal for Parasitology* **7**, 463–466.

DOBSON, C. & TANG, J. M. (1991). Genetic variation and host-parasite relations: *Nematospiroides dubius* in mice. *Journal of Parasitology* **77**, 884–889.

EDWARDS, A. J., BURT, J. S. & OGILVIE, B. M. (1971). The effect of immunity upon some enzymes of the parasitic nematode *Nippostrongylus brasiliensis*. *Parasitology* **62**, 339–347.

ELSE, K. J. & GRENCIS, R. K. (1999). Antibody-independent effector mechanisms in resistance to the intestinal nematode parasite *Trichuris muris*. *Infection and Immunity* **64**, 2950–2954.

ELSE, K. J. & WAKELIN, D. (1988). The effect of H-2 and non-H-2 genes on the expulsion of the nematode *Trichuris muris* from inbred and congenic mice. *Parasitology* **96**, 543–550.

FISHER, M. C. & VINEY, M. E. (1998). The population genetic structure of the facultatively sexual parasitic nematode *Strongyloides ratti* in wild rats. *Proceedings of the Royal Society of London B* **265**, 703–709.

FRASER, E. M. & KENNEDY, M. W. (1991). Heterogeneity in the expression of surface-exposed epitopes among larvae of *Ascaris lumbricoides*. *Parasite Immunology* **13**, 219–225.

GASSER, R. B. & NEWTON, S. E. (2000). Genomic and genetic research on bursate nematodes: significance, implications and prospects. *International Journal for Parasitology* **30**, 509–534.

GEMMILL, A. W., VINEY, M. E. & READ, A. F. (2000). The evolutionary ecology of host-specificity: experimental studies with *Strongyloides ratti*. *Parasitology* **120**, 429–437.

GIBBS, H. C. (1986). Hypobiosis in parasitic nematodes – an update. *Advances in Parasitology* **25**, 129–174.

GOYAL, P. K. & WAKELIN, D. (1993*a*). Influence of variation in host strain and parasite isolate on inflammatory and antibody responses to *Trichinella spiralis* in mice. *Parasitology* **106**, 371–378.

GOYAL, P. K. & WAKELIN, D. (1993*b*). Vaccination against *Trichinella spiralis* in mice using antigens from different isolates. *Parasitology* **107**, 311–317.

GOYAL, P. K., HERMANEK, J. & WAKELIN, D. (1994). Lymphocyte proliferation and cytokine production in mice infected with different geographical isolates of *Trichinella spiralis*. *Parasite Immunology* **16**, 105–110.

GRANT, W. N. & MASCORD, L. J. (1996). Beta-tubulin gene polymorphism and benzimidazole resistance in *Trichostrongylus colubriformis*. *International Journal for Parasitology* **26**, 71–77.

GRANT, W. N. & WHITTINGTON, G. E. (1994). Extensive DNA polymorphism within and between two strains of *Trichostrongylus colubriformis*. *International Journal for Parasitology* **24**, 719–725.

GRENCIS, R. K. (1996). T cell and cytokine basis of host variability in response to intestinal nematode infections. *Parasitology* **112**, S31–S37.

GRENCIS, R. K. & ENTWISTLE, G. M. (1997). Production of an interferon-gamma homologue by an intestinal nematode: functionally significant or interesting artefact? *Parasitology* **115**, S101–S106.

HALEY, J. A. (1966). Biology of the rat nematode *Nippostrongylus brasiliensis* (Travassos, 1914). III. Characteristics of *N. brasiliensis* after 30–120 serial passages in the Syrian hamster. *Journal of Parasitology* **52**, 98–108.

HALL, A. & HOLLAND, C. (2000). Geographical variation in *Ascaris lumbricoides* fecundity and its implications for helminth control. *Parasitology Today* **16**, 540–544.

HARNETT, W., DEEHAN, M. R., HOUSTON, K. M. & HARNETT, M. M. (1999). Immunomodulatory properties of a phosphorylcholine-containing secreted filarial glycoprotein. *Parasite Immunology* **21**, 601–608.

HAWDON, J. M., LI, T., ZHAN, B. & BLOUIN, M. S. (2001). Genetic structure of populations of the human hookworm, *Necator americanus*, in China. *Molecular Ecology* **10**, 1433–1437.

HOEKSTRA, R., CRIADO FORNELIO, A., FAKKELDIJ, J., BERGMAN, J. & ROOS, M. H. (1997). Microsatellites of the parasitic nematode *Haemonchus contortus*: polymorphism and linkage with a direct repeat. *Molecular and Biochemical Parasitology* **89**, 987–1007.

JENKINS, D. C. & PHILLIPSON, R. F. (1972). Evidence that the nematode *Nippostrongylus brasiliensis* can adapt to and overcome the effects of host immunity. *International Journal for Parasitology* **2**, 353–359.

KAPEL, C. M. O. (2000). Host diversity and biological characteristics of the *Trichinella* genotypes and their effect on transmission. *Veterinary Parasitology* **93**, 263–278.

KAPEL, C. M. O. & GAMBLE, H. R. (2000). Infectivity, persistence, and antibody response to domestic and sylvatic *Trichinella* spp. in experimentally infected pigs. *International Journal for Parasitology* **30**, 215–221.

KAPEL, C. M. O. (2001). Sylvatic and domestic *Trichinella* spp. in wild boars; infectivity, muscle larvae distribution, and antibody response. *Journal of Parasitology* **87**, 309–314.

KELLY, J. D., WHITLOCK, H. V., THOMPSON, H. G., HALL, C. A., MARTIN, I. C. A. & LE JAMBRE, L. F. (1978). Physiological characteristics of free-living and parasitic stages of *Haemonchus contortus*, susceptible or resistant to benzimidazole anthelmintics. *Research in Veterinary Science* **25**, 376–385.

KOYAMA, K. & ITO, Y. (1996). Comparative studies on immune responses to infection in susceptible B10.BR mice infected with different strains of the murine nematode parasite *Trichuris muris*. *Parasite Immunology* **18**, 257–263.

KOYAMA, K. & ITO, Y. (2001). Comparative studies on the levels of serum IgG1 and IgG2a in susceptible B10.BR mice infected with different strains of the intestinal nematode parasite *Trichuris muris*. *Parasitology Research* **87**, 570–572.

LA ROSA, G., MARUCCI, G., ZARLENGA, D. S. & POZIO, E. (2001). *Trichinella pseudospiralis* populations of the Palearctic region and their relationship with populations of the Nearctic and Australian regions. *International Journal for Parasitology* **31**, 297–305.

LA ROSA, G. & POZIO, E. (2000). Molecular investigation of African isolates of *Trichinella* reveals genetic polymorphism in *Trichinella nelsoni*. *International Journal for Parasitology* **30**, 663–667.

MACLEAN, J. M., LEWIS, D. & HOLMES, P. H. (1987). The pathogenesis of benzimidazole-resistant and benzimidazole-susceptible strains of *Trichostrongylus colubriformis* in the Mongolian gerbil (*Meriones unguiculatus*). *Journal of Helminthology* **61**, 179–189.

MAINGI, N., SCOTT, M. E. & PRICHARD, R. K. (1990). Effect of selection pressure for thiabendazole resistance on fitness of *Haemonchus contortus* in sheep. *Parasitology* **100**, 327–335.

MAIZELS, R. M., BUNDY, D. A. P., SELKIRK, M. E., SMITH, D. F. & ANDERSON, R. M. (1993). Immunological modulation and evasion by helminth parasites in human populations. *Nature* **365**, 797–805.

MALAKAUSKAS, A., KAPEL, C. M. O. & WEBSTER, P. (2000). Infectivity, persistence and serological response of nine *Trichinella* genotypes in rats. *Parasitology* **8**, S216–S222.

MALLET, S. & HOSTE, H. (1995). Physiology of two strains of *Trichostrongylus colubriformis* resistant and susceptible to thiabendazole and mucosal response of experimentally infected rabbits. *International Journal for Parasitology* **25**, 23–27.

MURRELL, K. D., LICHTENFELS, R. J., ZARLENGA, D. S. & POZIO, E. (2000). The systematics of the genus *Trichinella* with a key of species. *Veterinary Parasitology* **93**, 293–307.

NAGANO, I., WU, Z., MATSUO, A., POZIO, E. & TAKAHASHI, Y. (1999). Identification of *Trichinella* isolates by polymerase chain reaction–restriction fragment length polymorphism of the mitochondrial cytochrome c-oxidase submit I gene. *International Journal for Parasitology* **29**, 1113–1120.

NEWTON, S. E., MORRISH, L. E., MARTIN, P. J., MONTAGUE, P. E. & ROLPH, T. P. (1995). Protection against multiply drug-resistant and geographically distant strains of *Haemonchus contortus* by vaccination with H11, a gut membrane-derived protective antigen. *International Journal for Parasitology* **25**, 511–521.

OGILVIE, B. M. (1972). Protective immunity to *Nippostrongylus brasiliensis* in the rat. II. Adaptation by worms. *Immunology* **22**, 111–118.

PRICHARD, R. K. (2001). Genetic variability following selection of *Haemonchus contortus* with anthelmintics. *Trends in Parasitology* **17**, 445–453.

QUINNELL, R. J., BEHNKE, J. M. & KEYMER, A. E. (1991). Host specificity of and cross-immunity between two strains of *Heligmosomoides polygyrus*. *Parasitology* **102**, 419–427.

SEN, H. G. & SETH, D. (1967). Complete development of the human hookworm, *Necator americanus* in golden hamsters, *Mesocricetus auratus*. *Nature, London* **214**, 609–610.

SMITH, N. C. & BRYANT, C. (1986). The role of host-generated free radicals in helminth infections: *Nippostrongylus brasiliensis* and *Nematospiroides dubius* compared. *International Journal for Parasitology* **16**, 617–622

SOLOMON, M. S. & HALEY, J. A. (1966). Biology of the rat nematode *Nippostrongylus brasiliensus* (Travassos, 1914). V. Characteristics of *N. brasiliensis* after serial passage in the laboratory mouse. *Journal of Parasitology* **52**, 237–241.

SOLTYS, J., GOYAL, P. K. & WAKELIN, D. (1999). Cellular immune responses in mice infected with the intestinal nematode *Trichuris muris*. *Experimental Parasitology* **92**, 40–47.

STEWART, G. L. (1989). Biological and immunological characteristics of *Trichinella pseudospiralis*. *Parasitology Today* **5**, 344–349.

STEWART, G. L., MANN, M. A., UBELAKER, J. E., McCARTHY, J. L. & WOOD, B. G. (1988). A role for elevated plasma corticosterone in modulation of host response during infection with *Trichinella pseudospiralis*. *Parasite Immunology* **10**, 139–150.

SU, Z. & DOBSON, C. (1997). Genetic and immunological adaptation of *Heligmosomoides polygyrus* in mice. *International Journal for Parasitology* **27**, 653–663.

TANG, J., DOBSON, C. & McMANUS, D. P. (1995). Antigens in phenotypes of *Heligmosomoides polygyrus* raised selectively from different strains of mice. *International Journal for Parasitology* **25**, 847–852.

TELFORD, G., WHEELER, D. J., APPLEBY, P., BOWEN, J. G. & PRITCHARD, D. I. (1998). *Heligmosomoides polygyrus* immunomodulatory factor (IMF), targets T-lymphocytes. *Parasite Immunology* **20**, 601–611.

VINEY, M. E. (2001). Diversity in populations of parasitic nematodes and its significance. In *Parasitic Nematodes: Molecular Biochemistry and Immunology* (ed. Kennedy, M. W. & Harnett, W.), pp. 83–102. Wallingford, UK, CABI Publishing.

WAKELIN, D. (1973). The stimulation of immunity to *Trichuris muris* in mice exposed to low-level infections. *Parasitology* **66**, 181–189.

WAKELIN, D. & GOYAL, P. K. (1996). *Trichinella* isolates: parasite variability and host responses. *International Journal for Parasitology* **26**, 471–481.

WU, Z., NAGANO, I., POZIO, E. & TAKAHASHI, Y. (1999). Polymerase chain reaction-restriction fragment length polymorphism (PCR-RFLP) for the identification of *Trichinella* isolates. *Parasitology* **118**, 211–218.

ZARLENGA, D. S., CHUTE, M. B., MARTIN, A. & KAPEL, C. M. O. (1999). A multiplex PCR for unequivocal differentiation of all encapsulated and non-encapsulated genotypes of *Trichinella*. *International Journal for Parasitology* **29**, 1859–1867.

Schistosome genetic diversity: the implications of population structure as detected with microsatellite markers

J. CURTIS[2], R. E. SORENSEN[1] *and* D. J. MINCHELLA[1]*

[1] *Department of Biological Sciences, Purdue University, West Lafayette, IN 47907, USA*
[2] *Biology/Chemistry Section, Purdue University North Central, Westville, IN 46391, USA*

SUMMARY

Blood flukes in the genus *Schistosoma* are important human parasites in tropical regions. A substantial amount of genetic diversity has been described in populations of these parasites using molecular markers. We first consider the extent of genetic variation found in *Schistosoma mansoni* and some factors that may be contributing to this variation. Recently, though, attempts have been made to analyze not only the genetic diversity but how that diversity is partitioned within natural populations of schistosomes. Studies with non-allelic molecular markers (e.g. RAPDs and mtVNTRs) have indicated that schistosome populations exhibit varying levels of gene flow among component subpopulations. The recent characterization of microsatellite markers for *S. mansoni* provided an opportunity to study schistosome population structure within a population of schistosomes from a single Brazilian village using allelic markers. Whereas the detection of population structure depends strongly on the type of analysis with a mitochondrial marker, analyses with a set of seven microsatellite loci consistently revealed moderate genetic differentiation when village boroughs were used to define parasite subpopulations and greater subdivision when human hosts defined subpopulations. Finally, we discuss the implications that such strong population structure might have on schistosome epidemiology.

Key words: *Schistosoma mansoni*, population genetics, microsatellite.

GENETIC POLYMORPHISM IN SCHISTOSOMES

The interactions between hosts and parasites can be viewed as a co-evolutionary contest between the interacting species; numerous factors – both biotic (e.g. reciprocal genetic change) and abiotic (e.g. changes in the environment) – contribute to the outcome of the contest. Over the course of an infection, the host's genetic background and associated adaptive immune responses provide it with the means to avoid or combat parasite invasion. Conversely, the parasite's genotype may make the difference between successful propagation and elimination; this sort of co-evolutionary arms race is embodied in the 'Red Queen Hypothesis' (Van Valen, 1973). The genetic variation present in each of the respective populations can be viewed as the arsenal for each of the species involved in this never-ending contest.

An entire range of micro-evolutionary forces, which serve to alter the genetic composition of the competing populations, further complicates these interactions at the population level. Typically, parasites can only mate with conspecifics that have managed to coinfect their host, many of which could be closely related due to the transmission dynamics of the parasite's life cycle. The stochastic nature of parasite transmission dynamics may eliminate otherwise fit parasite genotypes from isolated populations. Finally, in the case of parasites of humans, hosts may take action that selects for parasite genotypes that are less susceptible to treatment with anti-parasitic drugs.

If the three major components of any host-parasite interaction are the abiotic environment, host genetics (whether human or snail host) and parasite genetics, it can easily be argued that the latter has been the least studied, even though it surely contributes to exposure outcomes as much as either of the other two. In our studies of schistosome parasites in Brazil, it is common to find households where there is significant among-host variation in infection intensity. While immunology and the environment certainly play a role in shaping such outcomes, parasite genetics is the other piece of the puzzle.

Our analyses of parasite genetics focus on *Schistosoma mansoni*, a trematode parasite of the mammalian blood system. These worms are responsible for human schistosomiasis, a debilitating disease in South America, the Caribbean, Africa and the Middle East. Schistosomes undergo sexual reproduction in human hosts and this presumably generates parasite genotypic diversity. The eggs laid by the female worm pass in the host's faeces and hatch in water to release miracidia. These free-swimming

* Corresponding author: Dennis J. Minchella, Department of Biological Sciences, Purdue University, West Lafayette, IN 47907, USA. Tel: 765-494-8188. Fax: 765-494-0876. E-mail: DennisM@purdue.edu

DOI: 10.1017/S0031182002002020 Printed in the United Kingdom

larvae must find and penetrate a freshwater snail (*Biomphalaria* spp.). The larval stages grow and multiply asexually within the snail (i.e. a single miracidium gives rise to many clonal offspring), emerging after several weeks as free-swimming cercariae that are infective to human hosts, thus completing the life cycle. A number of features of this life cycle may have interesting ramifications for the maintenance and distribution of parasite genetic diversity. Different schistosome genotypes may be brought together in space and time as: (1) male and female worms mate in the human host, (2) eggs representing the outcome of matings between different worm pairs are passed by defaecation of the host and (3) larval stages coinfect the same snail host and simultaneously release cercariae available for infection of human hosts.

In order to assess the relative role of various evolutionary forces on natural schistosome populations, we must determine the distributions of schistosome genotypes in these populations and their change over time. However, for populations of *S. mansoni*, little is known of the distribution of different parasite genotypes within and among populations (Curtis & Minchella, 2000). This dearth of knowledge has been due both to the lack of appropriate polymorphic genetic markers (Nadler, 1995) and to the difficulty in obtaining representative samples of schistosomes from natural populations. Infected intermediate hosts (*B. glabrata*) often occur at very low frequencies in the field and, because adult worms are sequestered within human hosts, they are not available for direct genetic characterization.

With the application of modern genetic methods, however, elucidation of the genetic structure of schistosome populations is gradually being realized. Using a highly polymorphic repetitive DNA marker, substantial genetic heterogeneity was detected among isolates from a single local site in Brazil (Minchella *et al.* 1994). High genotypic diversity has also been reported for parasites within rat definitive hosts in Guadeloupe using randomly amplified polymorphic DNA (RAPD) markers (Barral *et al.* 1996; Sire *et al.* 2001), though further studies are needed to compare this diversity with that found in humans. Schistosome genotypic diversity within molluscan host populations has also been characterized, often through infection of laboratory mice with cercariae shed from field-collected snails (Minchella, Sollenberger & deSousa, 1995; Dabo *et al.* 1997; Davies *et al.* 1999; Sire *et al.* 1999). These studies have sampled snail populations with a range of infection prevalences. Results support the hypothesis that a single intermediate host may harbour a number of different parasite genotypes and that these genotypes may represent a significant fraction of the parasite genotypic diversity at a collection site. As infection prevalence increases at a site, the distribution of the number of genotypes found within each snail becomes more uniform and thus the phenomenon of genotypic overdispersion appears to diminish (Eppert *et al.* 2002).

MEASURING POPULATION STRUCTURE IN SCHISTOSOMES

In studies of genetic variation in natural populations, the first step is to quantify the genetic variation present. While it is of value to know the variety of schistosomes that exist within a defined area, it would be even more advantageous to know how genotypes are distributed within and among parasite populations, and the epidemiological factors that determine these distributions. For schistosome populations infecting human hosts, it is possible to define subpopulations at a variety of hierarchical levels: all the worms within a patient, within all of the patients in a particular 'neighbourhood', within all of the 'neighbourhoods' that make up a village, within all of the villages that make up a region. The extent to which gene flow is restricted between these subpopulations determines the degree of population structure at each of the hierarchical levels (Wright, 1978; Slatkin, 1995).

Just as the schistosome life cycle affects genotype movement through biotic and abiotic environments, it also plays an important role in determining schistosome population structure. Infection foci for schistosomiasis must have three characteristics: (1) suitable snail habitat, (2) contamination of freshwater with host faeces and (3) areas where humans have contact with water containing infective parasite larvae. Areas that do not meet all of these criteria are not likely to become stable infection foci, and will serve as parasite population 'sinks' in the host-parasite landscape. Gene flow between parasite subpopulations will then depend on the rate at which schistosomes are transferred between infection foci, which in most cases, would depend on the movement of infected human hosts.

Two aspects of the snail host populations also contribute to the expectation of schistosome population structure. First, parasite infections are typically overdispersed in natural *Biomphalaria* populations, such that a minority of the snails in the population harbours the majority of the infections (summarized in Eppert *et al.* 2002). As described above, multiple genotypes of the parasite could then be transmitted through one or a few snails in a very localized area. Second, recent analyses of snail populations have indicated that these are themselves strongly subdivided, perhaps due to the ability of those snails to undergo self-fertilization (Langand *et al.* 1999). Strong subdivision of snail populations makes it more likely that local adaptations may develop, including resistance to the most common parasite genotypes. This could be followed by frequency-dependent selection such that hosts and parasites co-evolve on a short-term localized scale (Manning, Woolhouse & Ndamba, 1995; Dybdahl & Lively, 1996).

Early studies of population structure in schistosomes used isozymes to look for genetic differences between populations of *S. mansoni*: those that are transmitted through rodents, and populations that infected humans (Rollinson, 1986; Sene *et al.* 1997). More recently, other molecular markers have been employed for analyses of schistosome population subdivision. We have reported the population structure of schistosome parasites within 21 patients from a Brazilian village using a mitochondrial marker with a variable number of tandem repeats (mtVNTR), which is reviewed in more detail below (Curtis *et al.* 2001 *a*). Population structure of *Biomphalaria* snail hosts and adult schistosomes from rat definitive hosts have been compared on Guadeloupe using RAPD markers, with significant population structure being detected for both (Sire *et al.* 2001). The subdivision of *S. haematobium* in human patients has also been studied using RAPD markers (Brouwer *et al.* 2001). This latter analysis found little evidence of population structure, although most of the patient isolates came from schoolchildren who might have been infected at the same set of local transmission sites. When transmission sites are not widely separated (e.g. on separate watercourses), the expectation of subdivision due to geographic factors diminishes.

It is evident from these preliminary studies of schistosome population structure that the nature of the sampled host population will influence the amount of subdivision detected. Cross-sectional surveys of communities are more likely to reveal population structure than, for example, a population of schoolchildren. Studies of population structure in non-human vertebrates, while allowing for direct genetic characterization of adult worms, carry the caveat that schistosome transmission may be quite different in these systems due to patterns of host movement. In addition, the methods used in characterizing the schistosome genotypes may well influence the degree of population structure that is detected.

Population structure can be estimated by several different methods. For molecular analyses using markers such as RAPDs or DNA fingerprinting, genetic differences between individuals are generated in the form of presence/absence data (i.e. non-allelic data). Population structure is then inferred when different subpopulations exhibit varying frequencies for the different variants that make up each individuals profile (e.g. bands produced by gel electrophoresis). Estimating population structure with such data requires just the right amount of genetic polymorphism: insufficient levels do not provide sufficient resolution, but it is also possible that highly variable markers will make all individuals appear equally distant from one another, regardless of their true relationship (Estoup & Cornuet, 1999; J. Curtis, unpublished observations).

The *S. mansoni* mitochondrial genome contains a highly variable mtVNTR. The repeats in this polymorphic element, called pSM750, are 62 bp long, and the entire repeat region is flanked by restriction sites for the endonuclease *Rsa*I (Spotila, Rekosh & LoVerde, 1991). Each mitochondrial genome has the potential to carry a different number of these repeats and individual worms often contain multiple versions of the element (Curtis *et al.* 2001 *a*; Bieberich & Minchella, 2001), implying that there are a number of distinct mitochondrial haplotypes in the organelle population of each cell in the worm (i.e. the worms are heteroplasmic). By using pSM750 as a probe of genomic DNA from individual worms it is possible to detect a substantial amount of variation within a relatively small sample (Minchella *et al.* 1994, 1995), which in turn allows for the identification of differences between individual parasites within a single host. Population subdivision, based on the distribution of different haplotypes within subpopulations, can then be estimated using a class of hierarchical statistics designed for genetic data from organelles (C_{pt}: Lewontin, 1972; Birky, Fuerst & Murayama, 1989).

In order to utilize more advanced population genetic methods, schistosome population structure must be estimated using the observed number of heterozygotes among subpopulations; deficiencies in heterozygosity indicate potential cases of restricted gene flow or inbreeding (Wright, 1978; Slatkin, 1995). Thus, studies of population structure demand molecular markers that display allelism (Curtis & Minchella, 2000). Microsatellite loci – markers that meet these criteria – are DNA sequences characterized by a variable number of very short repeats (2–6 nucleotides each). Microsatellites have been effective tools for detecting genetic structure at limited spatial scales (Lougheed *et al.* 2000). A number of microsatellite loci have been described from the genome of *S. mansoni* (Durand, Sire & Théron, 2000; Curtis *et al.* 2001 *b*).

Allele frequency data for a population of worms can be used to calculate F_{ST} (Wright, 1969) by the method of Weir & Cockerham (1984), as well as ρ_{ST} (Michalakis & Excoffier, 1996), an unbiased estimate of the equivalent statistic (R_{ST}: Slatkin, 1995) that accounts for repeat length variation present in microsatellite data. Using the frequencies of the different alleles and the assumption that closely related alleles will have small size differences, population subdivision can be estimated for each of the loci; a final estimate can also be inferred across all loci. Higher values of F_{ST} (alternatively, ρ_{ST} for microsatellites, or C_{pt} for mtVNTR data) indicate greater differentiation of subpopulations (i.e. restricted gene flow), and thus more population structure.

FIELD STUDIES OF BRAZILIAN SCHISTOSOMES

In October 1997, we sampled parasite diversity in patients who live in the Brazilian village of Melquiades in the state of Minas Gerais. The prevalence of *S. mansoni* among the 800 citizens of the village was very high (75 %). The village consists of a collection of boroughs along several independent waterways with clusters of houses separated by 1–2 km of intervening agricultural land. Given this, it seemed unlikely that there could be a single intense focus of transmission. A total of 21 patients were sampled, representing each of the seven boroughs. The patient isolates were obtained by hatching miracidia from faecal samples and these miracidia were used to infect lab-reared snails. After 4–5 weeks, the cercariae emerging from these infected snails were used to infect mice. Once the schistosomes had matured, they were harvested from the mice by perfusion and used in the genetic analysis of each patient isolate.

DNA was extracted from 25–30 individual male schistosomes from each patient isolate (after Sorensen, Curtis & Minchella, 1998). As none of the molecular markers shows evidence of sex-linked inheritance, males are used exclusively because their larger bodies provide more DNA for the analysis. Worms were placed in 1·5 ml microcentrifuge tubes and pulverized on dry ice with a chilled pestle. The pestle was rinsed with a buffer containing 100 mM NaCl, 25 mM sucrose, 10 mM EDTA, and 2 % (m/v) SDS in 50 mM Tris, pH 8·0 (Brindley *et al.* 1989). This mixture was lysed at 65 °C for 30 min, then 8 M KOAc was added to a final concentration of 1 M, and lastly, it was chilled on ice for 30 min. Salts were removed from the mixture by spinning at 12000 rpm for 10 min. Standard ethanol precipitation practices (Sambrook, Fritsch & Maniatis, 1989) were used to pellet the DNA from the supernatant. Pellets were resuspended in 16 μl of water, with 13 μl being used in the DNA profiling analysis with the mtVNTR marker. The remaining 3 μl aliquot (approximately 150 ng of DNA) was diluted 1:10 with water and used in the microsatellite analysis.

The schistosomes comprising the patient isolates from Melquiades were first analysed by DNA profiling with the pSM750 mtVNTR marker (Curtis *et al.* 2001 *a*). Although this study analysed the subsequent generation after rearing through laboratory snails and mice, the marker's pattern of maternal inheritance (Bieberich & Minchella, 2001) allowed direct inference of mtVNTR haplotype diversity for the population within a single human host. On average, patients were infected with approximately 10 different schistosome genotypes (i.e. genotypes distinguished on the basis of distinct haplotype profiles), and very few genotypes were found in more than one patient isolate. We detected no correlation between the clustering of worm genotypes and any other epidemiological parameters (e.g. geography, patient age, patient sex, household or worm burden). Among the individual schistosomes, 72·5 % had heteroplasmic haplotype profiles, such that individual worms represented 46·9 % of the genetic variation present in the population. With so much of the variation described at the within-worm level of the population structure hierarchy, differentiation between patient isolates was low ($C_{pt} = 0{\cdot}060$) and subdivision between the seven boroughs was even less ($C_{pt} = 0{\cdot}025$). The apparent lack of population structure within schistosomes from Melquiades, despite a wealth of genotypic diversity, seemed to support the hypothesis that human hosts move throughout the village, acquiring infections from a variety of transmission sites, thereby creating the opportunity for different genotypes to mate.

Alternatively, a phenomenon such as an increased mutation rate or another feature of the genetic marker might be contributing to the apparent lack of population structure. In fact, we have evidence that the mutation rate for pSM750, which lies within the highly variable D-loop of the *S. mansoni* mitochondrial genome, may be as high as 10^{-1} events per generation (Bieberich & Minchella, 2001). This led us to suspect that haplotypes with an identical number of pSM750 repeats might not be the products of a common ancestor, but rather the result of a homoplasy-inducing mutational event (Estoup & Cornuet, 1999). This suspicion was further supported by the observation that many of the haplotypes fell within a narrow range of repeat sizes that appeared to be most common. Thus, the genotypes of many of these individual worms were comprised of one of the common haplotypes along with one or more of the less frequent haplotypes.

In an attempt to correct for the homoplasy present in the distribution of the common haplotypes, we recalculated the hierarchical statistics using only the 'rare' haplotypes (those present in 10 or fewer genotypes in the entire population) (Slatkin, 1985). Under this analysis, the within-worm component of the population's genetic variation dropped to 17 %, and much more of the variation was distributed within and among subpopulations (Table 3 in Curtis *et al.* 2001 *a*). Substantial differentiation was found among patient isolates ($C_{pt} = 0{\cdot}365$), and moderate subdivision was even detected among boroughs ($C_{pt} = 0{\cdot}138$). Thus, the two analyses using the mtVNTR as a marker provided conflicting results: little evidence of subdivision was detected when all haplotypes were considered, whereas rare haplotypes alone implied strong subdivision.

To resolve this ambiguity regarding the schistosome population structure in Melquiades, we reanalysed the schistosome isolates with a set of seven nuclear microsatellite loci as markers (Table 1;

Table 1. Microsatellite loci with repeat motif and allelic diversity

Locus	Reference	Repeat motif	No. of alleles detected
D28	Curtis *et al.* 2001*b*	GATA	14
D43	Curtis *et al.* 2001*b*	GATA	21
DA23	Curtis *et al.* 2001*b*	GATA	17
DO11	Curtis *et al.* 2001*b*	GATA	24
E2	L46951 in Durand *et al.* 2000	GAA	15
E4	R95529 in Durand *et al.* 2000	CAT	22
ED28	SMD28 in Durand *et al.* 2000	CAA	14

Durand *et al.* 2000; Curtis *et al.* 2001*b*) as these provide allelic data, so that levels of heterozygosity could be assessed. These loci were chosen on the basis of consistent and reproducible amplification under standard conditions (Curtis *et al.* 2001*b*).

Alleles from at least five of seven loci were scored for a total of 295 worms. For four of the 21 patient isolates, fewer than 10 worms could be scored at any of the loci. These isolates were omitted from the analysis, and while all seven boroughs were still represented, some were represented by a single patient isolate. Also, prior to the calculation of allele frequencies, 29 worms were removed from the analysis on the basis of redundancy with other worms in the data-set from the same patient. The assumption underlying this removal was that if worms from the same patient isolate were indistinguishable with 7 microsatellite loci, then they were most likely clonal siblings produced asexually during passage through laboratory snails and should only be counted once to avoid pseudo-replication. Interestingly, the occurrence of clonal siblings within samples from patient isolates was relatively uncommon. A single worm pair within a patient could generate large numbers of multi-locus microsatellite genotypes among their offspring, and it seemed that many of these different offspring genotypes occurred in our sample. Because microsatellite loci are assumed to be selectively neutral, it is assumed in our analysis that any loss of genotypes that may occur during the laboratory passage is random (i.e. no selection occurs).

The schistosome population sample from Melquiades exhibited considerable allelic diversity at all of the loci sampled (mean = 18·9 alleles/locus). Observed heterozygosities were calculated at several different levels: at each locus within each patient isolate, across all loci within each patient isolate, across all patient isolates for each locus, and averaged for all loci across all worms within each isolate. The average within-worm heterozygosity values for each of the isolates ranged between 0·34 and 0·69 (Table 2), and were not correlated with the number of maternal genotypes previously estimated from each patient isolate using pSM750 ($R^2 = 0{\cdot}08$, $P = 0{\cdot}29$). This would seem to imply that the level of heterozygosity in the offspring was independent of the genetic diversity of worm pairs that were producing the eggs in the patient.

Heterozygosities at each of the loci ranged between 0·33 and 0·73 (Table 2). There was no correlation between the number of alleles detected at a locus and the average heterozygosity at that locus ($R^2 = 0{\cdot}15$, $P = 0{\cdot}39$). Worms were heterozygous at an average of 57% (S.D. 19%) of their loci. Heterozygosities (at all loci scored) within each of the 17 patient isolates ranged between 0·33 and 0·69.

Values for F_{ST} and ρ_{ST} were calculated using 'Genepop on the Web' (Rousset & Raymond, 1995; as implemented at http://wbiomed.curtin.edu.au/genepop). The value for Wright's F_{ST} varied between loci (Table 3). F_{ST} values were higher when individual hosts were treated as subpopulations (F_{ST}, all loci = 0·11) than when boroughs were treated as subpopulations (F_{ST}, all loci = 0·06) (paired *t* test, D.F. = 12, $P < 0{\cdot}01$). The values for ρ_{ST} also varied across loci (Table 3), and were again higher when human hosts were used to define the subpopulations (ρ_{ST}, all loci = 0·19) than when boroughs were used to define the subpopulations (ρ_{ST}, all loci = 0·07) (paired *t* test, D.F. = 12, $P = 0{\cdot}01$). Because they are both measures of population structure, values for ρ_{ST} and F_{ST} were also compared under the two hierarchical regimes. F_{ST} and ρ_{ST} did not differ significantly either when hosts were used as subpopulations (paired *t* test, D.F. = 12, $P = 0{\cdot}25$) or when boroughs were used (paired *t* test, D.F. = 12, $P = 0{\cdot}15$).

The values for F_{ST} and ρ_{ST} indicate that there is some degree of population structure for the schistosomes from this single village. While the overall values (Table 3) indicate that gene flow is restricted between some or all of the subpopulations, this single measurement does not indicate whether all of the subpopulations are equally differentiated, or whether parasites from some areas are more genetically distinct than others. In order to examine the extent of separation between parasites from the different boroughs, we calculated F_{ST} for all possible pairs of boroughs. Recalling that F_{ST} is inversely related to gene flow, these data can be used to infer which boroughs are experiencing migration of schistosomes to/from other boroughs. The results of this analysis (Fig. 1) indicate that certain boroughs (e.g. I, II and III) are essentially undifferentiated, while others (e.g. IV and V) are much more distinct. The observation that parasites in the 'upstream' boroughs are closely related, while those 'downstream' appear to be more independent, would seem to imply that schistosome gene flow is not strongly influenced by movement of aquatic larval forms or

Table 2. Observed heterozygosity (H_o) values by locus and patient isolate. The numbers in parentheses indicate the number of worms for which that locus was scored in that patient isolate

Patient ID	D28	D43	DA23	DO11	E2	E4	ED28	Within-patient H_o	Average within-worm H_o
M68	0·77 (30)	0·67 (30)	0·53 (30)	0·67 (27)	0·61 (28)	0·63 (27)	0·43 (30)	0·614	0·613
M71	0·90 (10)	0·50 (10)	0·70 (10)	0·78 (9)	0·50 (8)	0·78 (9)	0·10 (10)	0·606	0·614
M77	0·75 (8)	0·25 (8)	0·33 (3)	0·38 (8)	0·00 (3)	0·40 (5)	0·00 (8)	0·326	0·338
M82	1·00 (5)	1·00 (6)	0·67 (6)	0·50 (6)	0·25 (4)	0·67 (6)	0·33 (6)	0·641	0·639
M165	0·44 (9)	0·56 (9)	0·56 (9)	1·00 (9)	0·20 (5)	0·57 (7)	0·67 (9)	0·596	0·602
M168	0·57 (27)	0·23 (22)	0·38 (21)	0·95 (22)	0·95 (19)	0·45 (22)	0·18 (22)	0·523	0·536
M180	0·92 (13)	0·77 (13)	0·62 (13)	0·31 (13)	0·80 (10)	0·46 (13)	0·46 (13)	0·614	0·606
M181	0·86 (21)	0·87 (23)	0·39 (18)	0·78 (23)	0·31 (16)	0·40 (20)	0·22 (23)	0·563	0·556
M182	0·91 (22)	0·86 (22)	0·50 (22)	0·48 (21)	0·68 (22)	0·36 (22)	0·55 (22)	0·621	0·620
M253	0·80 (20)	0·55 (20)	0·55 (20)	0·85 (20)	0·65 (20)	1·00 (20)	0·45 (20)	0·693	0·693
M263	0·60 (25)	0·64 (25)	0·56 (25)	0·86 (21)	0·48 (21)	0·83 (24)	0·44 (25)	0·627	0·622
M326	0·80 (20)	0·65 (20)	0·55 (20)	0·80 (20)	0·79 (19)	0·45 (20)	0·15 (20)	0·597	0·589
M433	0·50 (23)	0·61 (23)	0·30 (23)	0·64 (22)	0·52 (23)	0·40 (20)	0·55 (22)	0·513	0·507
M434	0·29 (7)	0·33 (6)	0·75 (8)	0·50 (8)	0·50 (8)	0·40 (5)	0·56 (7)	0·490	0·521
M531	0·82 (17)	0·76 (17)	0·29 (17)	0·44 (16)	0·40 (15)	0·53 (17)	0·31 (16)	0·513	0·523
M626	0·79 (19)	0·79 (19)	0·47 (19)	0·26 (19)	0·53 (19)	0·28 (18)	0·05 (19)	0·390	0·383
M628	0·65 (20)	0·65 (20)	0·60 (20)	0·90 (20)	0·25 (20)	0·95 (20)	0·15 (20)	0·593	0·586
Within-locus H_o	0·73	0·65	0·50	0·68	0·55	0·57	0·33		

Table 3. Population subdivision by human host and borough

	Hosts as subpopulations		Boroughs as subpopulations	
Locus	F_{ST}	ρ_{ST}	F_{ST}	ρ_{ST}
D28	0·08	0·12	0·04	0·05
D43	0·09	0·18	0·03	0·02
DA23	0·14	0·10	0·05	0·04
DO11	0·10	0·08	0·07	0·06
E2	0·07	0·06	0·03	0·04
E4	0·10	0·07	0·09	0·06
ED28	0·11	0·18	0·05	0·05
All	0·11	0·19	0·06	0·07

snails, but rather a product of human movement. In fact, human residents in the upstream boroughs frequent the same areas (school, church, etc.), but have little occasion to travel to the more distant boroughs. These results demonstrate that a substantial amount of genetic differentiation can develop in schistosome populations, even over small geographic scales, and that the micro-evolutionary forces that produce such separation are most likely to be countered by migration facilitated by human hosts. Further analyses are needed to examine the persistence of this pattern of differentiation over greater geographic scales (i.e. among different villages and geographic regions).

Thus, the microsatellite analysis of schistosome isolates collected from human hosts in the Brazilian village of Melquiades revealed an impressive amount of allelic diversity even though all of the patients came from a fairly small geographic area (< 50 km^2). For all of the seven loci used in this study, the number of different alleles detected at Melquiades exceeded the diversity reported from sample populations when those loci were characterized (Durand *et al.* 2000; Curtis *et al.* 2001*b*). The amount of allelic diversity present, in combination with the fact that many of the rare alleles at the extreme of the size range were found in a single patient isolate, provided ideal conditions for an examination of population structure. The hierarchical statistics for schistosomes from Melquiades indicate moderate genetic differentiation among the subpopulations in the seven boroughs and greater genetic differentiation between the schistosomes that comprise an individual human host's infection. The extent to which these microsatellite data corroborate the results of the rare haplotype analysis seems to confirm that the common haplotypes are generating 'noise' that might obscure the detection of population subdivision, and suggests that there is reduced gene flow among the subpopulations that comprise the schistosome population of Melquiades.

IMPLICATIONS OF POPULATION STRUCTURE

It has been suggested that the high genetic diversity of schistosomes within individual vertebrate hosts may reflect the tendency of these hosts to move about the environment, sampling a number of transmission sites, thereby becoming 'genetic mixing bowls' for the parasites (Curtis & Minchella, 2000). However,

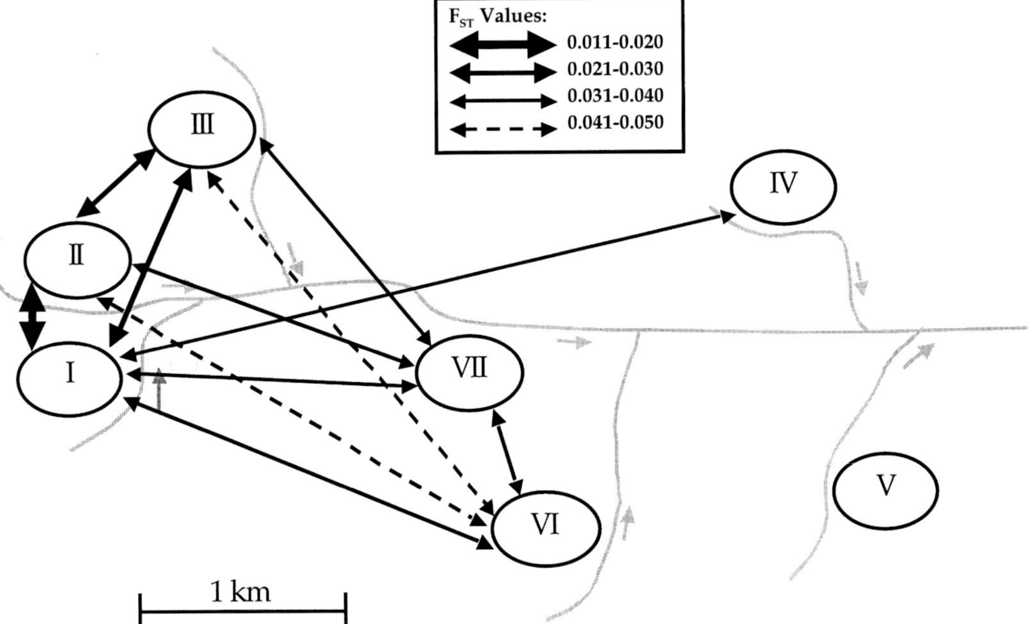

Fig 1. Schematic representation of schistosome gene flow within the Brazilian village of Melquiades. The relative positions of the seven boroughs of the village that were sampled are shown. The thickness of the arrow connecting a pair of boroughs reflects the amount of gene flow between their respective schistosome populations. More gene flow between boroughs would result in a lower value for F_{ST}. Lack of a connection between boroughs indicates that those boroughs are at least moderately differentiated ($F_{ST} > 0{\cdot}05$). Major watercourses and direction of flow are shown in grey.

patients in Melquiades appear to be 'under-sampling' the range of schistosome genetic variation in the village. Two alternative explanations are possible: either (1) patients are sampling a large number of sites throughout the village, but because of the stochasticity of infection processes, only a subset of the genotypes are able to successfully infect each patient; or (2) patients are more likely to be infected at transmission sites close to their home, with a rapidly diminishing probability of infection at more distant sites. The latter explanation would appear to be supported by the following two observations. First, a majority of the contact that humans have with cercariae-contaminated water is likely to occur within a short distance of their home (e.g. while performing household duties for adults, while playing for children). This pattern of infection is reflected in the higher similarity of parasite genotypes from adjacent boroughs (Fig. 1). Second, the subpopulations within patients are even more strongly differentiated than the subpopulations of their respective boroughs. Thus, it would appear that patients are not even sampling their local area exhaustively.

If schistosome populations are strongly subdivided, along with populations of the snail intermediate hosts, then the conditions are right for localized adaptation between the parasites and their snail (and potentially, even human) hosts. The results presented here, along with those from other recent studies, indicate that the potential for local adaptation is present. What remains unknown are the mechanisms involved, the rate at which this co-evolution could occur, and the types of genes that are likely to be affected by the selective pressures of co-adaptation. Such local adaptation cannot be examined with the same markers that are used in studies of population structure, as these markers are, by necessity, selectively neutral.

The widespread application of a large set of microsatellite markers will not only contribute to a more complete understanding of schistosome biology; a number of important issues in the study of epidemiology will also become more tractable for study. For instance, schistosome populations that exhibit a polymorphism in response to chemotherapy (Feng, Curtis & Minchella, 2001) might also have demonstrable genetic differentiation at one or more microsatellite loci. At this point, these loci cease to become neutral genetic markers appropriate for population genetic studies; however, these loci would then become useful markers for resistance and might aid in genomic searches for resistance genes. Thus, more studies of natural populations with microsatellite markers are required to further our understanding of schistosome genetic structure and transmission dynamics.

Recent years have seen significant elucidation of the extent and distribution of genetic variation in natural *S. mansoni* populations. Thus far, the data depict only static moments in what is one of the most dynamic micro-evolutionary processes. The current studies need to be extended to quantify the magnitude of parasite genetic change over time and space. Long-term epidemiological studies in several natural host-parasite systems will allow for accurate modeling of infection and transmission dynamics. Estimates of parasite gene flow, derived from genetic analyses of the parasite sub-populations across many levels of the population structure hierarchy, have the potential to further our understanding of a number of disease processes: how super-infection (i.e. co-infection by multiple genotypes) may affect pathogenicity or the evolution of virulence, the genetic consequences of various control strategies for the parasite population, and the distribution of variation for genetic markers relevant to vaccine development throughout the range of this cosmopolitan parasite.

ACKNOWLEDGEMENTS

We would like to thank L. A. Fraga, C. P. de Souza, and R. Correa-Oliveira for assistance with our field studies in Brazil. This work received financial support from the National Institutes of Health (NIH RO1-A1 42768) and the National Science Foundation (DMS-9974389).

REFERENCES

BARRAL, V., MORAND, S., POINTIER, J. P. & THÉRON, A. (1996). Distribution of schistosome genetic diversity within naturally infected *Rattus rattus* detected by RAPD markers. *Parasitology* **113**, 511–517.

BIEBERICH, A. A. & MINCHELLA, D. J. (2001). Mitochondrial inheritance in *Schistosoma mansoni*: mtVNTR mutation produces noise on top of the signal. *Journal of Parasitology* **87**, 1011–1015.

BIRKY, C. W. JR., FUERST, P. & MARUYAMA, T. (1989). Organelle gene diversity under migration, mutation, and drift: equilibrium expectations, approach to equilibrium, effects of heteroplasmic cells, and comparison to nuclear genes. *Genetics* **121**, 613–627.

BRINDLEY, P. J., LEWIS, F. A., MCCUTCHAN, T. F., BUEDING, E. & SHER, A. (1989). A genomic change associated with the development of resistance to hycanthone in *Schistosoma mansoni*. *Molecular and Biochemical Parasitology* **36**, 243–252.

BROUWER, K. C., NDHLOVU, P., MUNATSI, A. & SHIFF, C. J. (2001). Genetic diversity of a population of *Schistosoma haematobium* derived from schoolchildren in east central Zimbabwe. *Journal of Parasitology* **87**, 762–769.

CURTIS, J., FRAGA, L. A., DE SOUZA, C. P., CORREA-OLIVEIRA, R. & MINCHELLA, D. J. (2001 *a*). Widespread heteroplasmy in schistosomes makes a mtVNTR marker 'nearsighted'. *Journal of Heredity* **92**, 248–253.

CURTIS, J. & MINCHELLA, D. J. (2000). Schistosome population genetic structure: when clumping worms is not just splitting hairs. *Parasitology Today* **16**, 68–71.

CURTIS, J., SORENSEN, R. E., PAGE, L. K. & MINCHELLA, D. J. (2001 *b*). Microsatellite loci in the human blood fluke *Schistosoma mansoni* and their utility for other schistosome species. *Molecular Ecology Notes* **1**, 143–145.

DABO, A., DURAND, P., MORAND, S., DIAKITE, M., LANGAND, J., IMBERT-ESTABLET, D., DOUMBO, O. & JOURDANE, J. (1997). Distribution and genetic diversity of *Schistosoma haematobium* within its bulinid intermediate hosts in Mali. *Acta Tropica* **66**, 15–26.

DAVIES, C. M., WEBSTER, J. P., KRUGER, O., MUNATSI, A., NDAMBA, J. & WOOLHOUSE, M. E. J. (1999). Host-parasite population genetics: a cross-sectional comparison of *Bulinus globosus* and *Schistosoma haematobium*. *Parasitology* **119**, 295–302.

DURAND, P., SIRE, C. & THÉRON, A. (2000). Isolation of microsatellite markers in the digenetic trematode *Schistosoma mansoni* from Guadeloupe island. *Molecular Ecology* **9**, 997–998.

DYBDAHL, M. F. & LIVELY, C. M. (1996). The geography of coevolution: comparative population structures for a snail and its trematode parasite. *Evolution* **50**, 2264–2275.

EPPERT, A., LEWIS, F. A., GRZYWACZ, C., COURA-FILHO, P. & MINCHELLA, D. J. (2002). Distribution of schistosome infections in molluscan hosts at different levels of parasite prevalence. *Journal of Parasitology* **88**, 232–236.

ESTOUP, A. & CORNUET, J. (1999). Microsatellite evolution: inferences from population data. In *Microsatellites: Evolution and Applications* (ed. Goldstein, D. B. & Schlötterer, C.), pp. 49–65. New York, Oxford University Press.

FENG, Z., CURTIS, J. & MINCHELLA, D. J. (2001). The influence of drug treatment on the maintenance of schistosome genetic diversity. *Journal of Mathematical Biology* **43**, 52–68.

LANGAND, J., THÉRON, A., POINTIER, J. P., DELAY, B. & JOURDANE, J. (1999). Population structure of *Biomphalaria glabrata*, intermediate host of *Schistosoma mansoni* in Guadeloupe Island, using RAPD markers. *Journal of Molluscan Studies* **65**, 425–433.

LEWONTIN, R. C. (1972). The apportionment of human diversity. *Evolutionary Biology* **6**, 381–398.

LOUGHEED, S. C., GIBBS, H. L., PRIOR, K. A. & WEATHERHEAD, P. J. (2000). A comparison of RAPD versus microsatellite DNA markers in population studies of the massasauga rattlesnake. *Journal of Heredity* **91**, 458–463.

MANNING, S. D., WOOLHOUSE, M. E. J. & NDAMBA, J. (1995). Geographic compatibility of the freshwater snail *Bulinus globosus* and schistosomes from the Zimbabwe highveld. *International Journal for Parasitology* **25**, 37–42.

MICHALAKIS, Y. & EXCOFFIER, L. (1996). A generic estimation of population subdivision using distances between alleles with special reference for microsatellite loci. *Genetics* **142**, 1060–1064.

MINCHELLA, D. J., LEWIS, F. A., SOLLENBERGER, K. M. & WILLIAMS, J. A. (1994). Genetic diversity of *Schistosoma mansoni*: quantifying strain heterogeneity using a polymorphic DNA element. *Molecular and Biochemical Parasitology* **68**, 307–313.

MINCHELLA, D. J., SOLLENBERGER, K. M. & DE SOUZA, C. P. (1995). Distribution of schistosome genetic diversity within molluscan intermediate hosts. *Parasitology* **111**, 217–220.

NADLER, S. (1995). Microevolution and the genetic structure of parasite populations. *Journal of Parasitology* **81**, 395–403.

ROLLINSON, D. (1986). *Schistosoma mansoni* from naturally infected *Rattus rattus* in Guadeloupe: identification, prevalence and enzyme polymorphism. *Parasitology* **93**, 39–53.

ROUSSET, F. & RAYMOND, M. (1995). Testing heterozygote excess and deficiency. *Genetics* **140**, 1413–1419.

SAMBROOK, J., FRITSCH, E. F. & MANIATIS, T. (1989). *Molecular Cloning: A Laboratory Manual*. New York, Cold Spring Harbor Laboratory Press.

SENE, M., BRÉMOND, P., HERVE, J. P., SOUTHGATE, V. R., SELLIN, B., MARCHAND, B. & DUPLANTIER, J. M. (1997). Comparison of human and murine isolates of *Schistosoma mansoni* from Richard-Toll, Senegal, by isoelectric focusing. *Journal of Helminthology* **71**, 175–181.

SIRE, C., DURAND, P., POINTIER, J. P. & THÉRON, A. (1999). Genetic diversity and recruitment pattern of *Schistosoma mansoni* in a *Biomphalaria glabrata* snail population: a field study using random-amplified polymorphic DNA markers. *Journal of Parasitology* **85**, 436–441.

SIRE, C., LANGAND, J., BARRAL, V. & THÉRON, A. (2001). Parasite (*Schistosoma mansoni*) and host (*Biomphalaria glabrata*) genetic diversity: population structure in a fragmented landscape. *Parasitology* **122**, 545–554.

SLATKIN, M. (1985). Rare alleles as indicators of gene flow. *Evolution* **39**, 53–65.

SLATKIN, M. (1995). Gene flow and the geographic structure of natural populations. *Science* **236**, 787–792.

SORENSEN, R. E., CURTIS, J. & MINCHELLA, D. J. (1998). Intraspecific variation in the rDNA ITS loci of 37-collar-spined echinostomes from North America: implications for sequence-based diagnoses and phylogenetics. *Journal of Parasitology* **84**, 992–997.

SPOTILA, L. D., REKOSH, D. M. & LOVERDE, P. T. (1991). Polymorphic repeated DNA element in the genome of *Schistosoma mansoni*. *Molecular and Biochemical Parasitology* **48**, 117–120.

VAN VALEN, L. (1973). A new evolutionary law. *Evolutionary Theory* **1**, 1–30.

WEIR, B. S. & COCKERHAM, C. C. (1984). Estimating F-statistics for the analysis of population structure. *Evolution* **38**, 1358–1370.

WRIGHT, S. (1969). *Evolution and the Genetics of Populations, Volume 2. The Theory of Gene Frequencies*. Chicago, University of Chicago Press.

WRIGHT, S. (1978). *Evolution and the Genetics of Populations, Volume 4. Variability Within and Among Natural Populations*. Chicago, University of Chicago Press.

The epidemiological consequences of optimisation of the individual host immune response

G. F. MEDLEY

Ecology & Epidemiology Group, Department of Biological Sciences, University of Warwick, Coventry CV4 7AL

SUMMARY

We present a simple unscaled, quantitative framework that addresses the optimum use of resources throughout a host's lifetime based on continuous exposure to parasites (rather than evolutionary, genetically explicit trade-offs). The principal assumptions are that a host's investment of resources in growth increases its survival and reproduction, and that increasing parasite burden reduces survival. The host reproductive value is maximised for a given combination of rates of parasite exposure, host resource acquisition and pathogenicity, which results in an optimum parasite burden (for the host). Generally, results indicate that the optimum resource allocation is to tolerate some parasite infection. The lower the resource acquisition, the lower the proportion of resources that should be devoted to immunity, i.e. the higher the optimum parasite burden. Increases in pathogenicity result in reduced optimum parasite burdens, whereas increases in exposure result in increasing optimum parasite burdens. Simultaneous variation in resource acquisition, pathogenicity and exposure within a community of hosts results in overdispersed parasite burdens, with the degree of heterogeneity decreasing as mean burden increases. The relationships between host condition and parasite burden are complicated, and could potentially confound data analysis. Finally, the value of this approach for explaining epidemiological patterns, immunological processes and the possibilities for further work are discussed.

Key words: Epidemiology, immunity, mathematical models, parasites, resource allocation.

INTRODUCTION

Evolutionary success is built on reproduction and survival – all other physiological mechanisms are designed to increase these and, therefore, fitness. The immune system is no exception. A simplistic view is that, by definition, parasitic infection reduces fitness of the host, and that an immune response nullifies or reduces this effect by killing parasites. However, immunity and immune responses occur at a cost of resources (such as energy and protein), and resources are limited, so there will be a trade-off between mounting an immunological response and reduction in fitness (Behnke, Barnard & Wakelin, 1992; Sheldon & Velhurst, 1996; Lochmiller & Deerenberg, 2000; Read & Allen, 2000). There is an increasing number of experimental examples placing the immune response within an ecological, epidemiological and evolutionary context (e.g. Boots & Begon, 1993; Gustafsson *et al.* 1994; Kraaijeveld & Godfray, 1997; Fellowes, Kraaijeveld & Godfray, 1998; Moret & Schmid-Hempel, 2000). If immunity is constrained by resource acquisition, then a complex relationship between, for example, nutrition and immunity to parasites is to be expected (e.g. Coop & Kyriazakis, 1999). Generally, reduced nutritional intake (or acquisition) will reduce resilience to infection and/or disease, although the effect may be subtle and depend on sub-optimal nutrition rather than malnutrition (Michael & Bundy, 1992*a*, *b*; Petkevicius *et al.* 1995). Similarly, as behaviour is a determinant of fitness, there is an intimate link between immunity and behaviour (Barnard *et al.* 1997).

An enduring subject in parasite epidemiology is the heterogeneity observed in parasite burdens, and understanding the roles of variation in exposure and immune competence (Quinnell, Medley & Keymer, 1990; Bundy & Medley, 1992; Hudson & Dobson, 1995). The distribution of parasites in a population of hosts is a dynamic entity (Anderson & Medley, 1985), with the controlling mechanisms predominately operating at the level of individual hosts. Longitudinal observations demonstrate that individual hosts have a tendency to reacquire relatively similar parasite burdens following expulsion chemotherapy, i.e. hosts appear to be predisposed to high or low burdens (e.g. Keymer & Pagel, 1990; Chan, Bundy & Kan, 1994*a*). Genetic influences appear to be important, but not over-riding (Chan, Bundy & Kan, 1994*b*; Williams-Blangero *et al.* 1999).

Host response to parasitic infection is recognized to depend on the pattern of exposure (e.g. Roepstorff *et al.* 1997). In recent experiments using *Ascaris suum* in pigs subject to a continuous, 'natural' exposure, Boes *et al.* (1998) showed that, in addition to predisposition, continued exposure results in a decrease in heterogeneity caused by a reduction in burdens of those heavily infected individuals and an increase in prevalence as pigs with zero burdens acquire small numbers. Further, the distribution of *A. suum* in litters of piglets shows reduced het-

Tel: +44 (0) 24 7652 4456. Fax: +44 (0) 24 7652 4619.
E-mail: graham.medley@warwick.ac.uk

Parasitology (2002), **125**, S61–S70.
DOI: 10.1017/S0031182002002354 Printed in the United Kingdom

erogeneity if sows are exposed (Boes *et al.* 1999). The results of cross-suckling strongly suggest that the reduction in heterogeneity is due to immunomodulation, i.e. piglets suckling from infected sows show the same response to challenge infection regardless of the infection status of their natural mother. Taken together, these experiments provide evidence that exposure to infection can increase parasite burden, and that this increased parasitism can be mediated by the immune response, i.e. the immune system is 'allowing' more parasites. Note that this effect of immunomodulation can only be seen in groups of hosts – the mean and individual burdens are not necessarily altered by exposure, but the variation within a group is reduced. Further insight into the interaction between heterogeneity and exposure is given by analysis of observational data that demonstrates that the degree of heterogeneity is decreased within a community/group of hosts as parasite prevalence increases (Guyatt *et al.* 1990, 1994; Lwambo, Bundy & Medley, 1992; Medley *et al.* 1993; Coates, Roepstorff & Medley, unpublished).

Thus, one should not expect, *ceteris paribus*, that increasing parasite challenge will lead to increased immune effectiveness either within individuals, or within populations. Epidemiological patterns of infection and disease observed at the population level are a manifestation of effects occurring within individual hosts that might be very different from an average effect. For example, the relationship between some measure of health (e.g. anaemia) and parasite burden, is complicated by the fact that individuals are controlling both anaemia and parasite burdens in order to maximise other variables, e.g. survival.

The interaction between resource acquisition, parasites, immunity and fitness is a quantitative problem that can be addressed through application of mathematical models. Previous theoretical work has largely concentrated on consideration of co-evolution of hosts and parasites, i.e. the dynamics of genetically controlled traits of susceptibility/resistance and pathogenicity (e.g. Antonovics & Thrall, 1994; Bowers, Boots & Begon, 1994; Kaitala, Heino & Getz, 1997). The results generally show that genetically controlled susceptibility to infection (and morbidity and mortality) can be maintained in a population if the fitness cost of resistance is great compared to the disease cost of susceptibility. Taking a game theory approach, van Baalen (1998) showed that the optimum resource allocation to immunity in a homogeneous population of hosts is determined by parasite characteristics such as virulence.

Here, we consider the problem from the viewpoint of an individual host, addressing physiological, rather than evolutionary (genetic), processes. The host is followed through age: how should it optimally distribute resources between reproduction, survival and immunity to maximise fitness? A similar framework has been used to consider both development of acquired immune response (Woolhouse, 1992) and development of disease and optimal age for infection control (Medley & Bundy, 1996). Initially, we simply illustrate the point that constrained resources can compromise immunity. The model is then used to demonstrate that this approach can potentially explain numerous ecological and immunological observations.

MODEL FRAMEWORK

The model is based on an individual host considered over age, a. Exposure to the parasite (measured as the rate of infection) is assumed not to depend directly on the parasite burden within the host. Resources can be used either to control the parasite burden (immunity) or for investment in growth or reproduction. The current parasite burden, (previous) investment and immunological response determine survival of the host. Age and (previous) investment determine reproductive output. Here the term 'immunity' is used to refer to host processes that constrain the parasite population, are adaptive and elicited by exposure to the parasite.

Resources are acquired at a constant rate, R, and are then partitioned between three competing requirements: growth, reproduction and immunity, designated f_g, f_r and f_i respectively, so that $f_g+f_r+f_i = R$. The growth component is used to increase the size of the individual, $g(a)$. Note that size is being used as a proxy for investment, i.e. using resources now to increase future survival and reproduction. We assume a standard growth rate equation:

$$\frac{dg}{da} = f_g\, g(1-g), \tag{1}$$

giving a nominal maximum size of unity, and using an initial size of 0·01. The parasite population, $p(a)$, is modelled as an immigration–death process (Bundy & Medley, 1992), where immigration (establishment) is reduced according to the resources devoted to immunity:

$$\frac{dp}{da} = \Lambda \exp(-3f_i) - \mu p. \tag{2}$$

The rates of establishment and death of the parasite population are Λ and μ, respectively. The exponential function is chosen arbitrarily such that for $f_i = 1$ the establishment rate of parasites is reduced to 95 % of its unconstrained level. We set $\mu = 1$ so that the maximum parasite burden when the rate of infection is constant is equal to Λ.

Resources are partitioned by first removing that component required for immunity:

$$f_i = \alpha R \frac{p}{1+p}. \tag{3}$$

This function increases as the parasite population increases up to a maximum, αR. The parameter α is

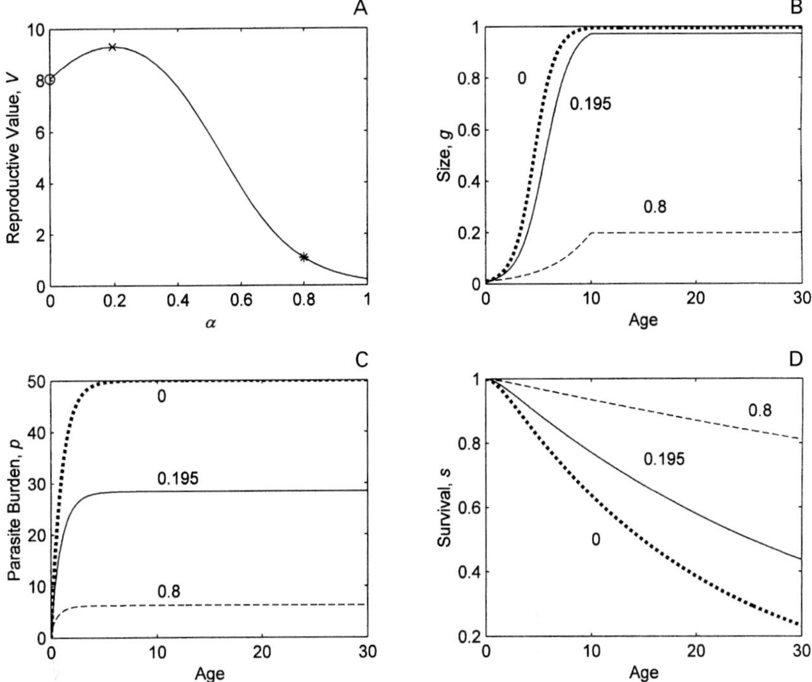

Fig. 1. Example output from the model (eqns 1–8). (a) The relationship between reproductive value (V) and maximum immunity resource (α). The three marked values coincide with lines in other panels. (b) The size (g) as a function of age for the three values of α (○: $\alpha = 0$, dotted line; x: $\alpha = 0{\cdot}195$, solid line; $*$: $\alpha = 0{\cdot}8$, dashed line). Note that nil investment in immunity (dotted line) results in maximal growth. (c) The parasite burden over age for the same values of α. The equilibrium parasite burden is reduced by increased resource allocation to immunity. (d) The survivorship curves over age for the same values of α. Other parameter values are $R = 1$, $\Lambda = 50$, $\beta = 1$.

important as it denotes the maximum proportion of resources a host will devote to controlling the (current) parasite population as opposed to investing in growth and reproduction. The resources remaining after immunity are used either for growth or reproduction, and for convenience, we choose an age of sexual maturity, $w = 10$, below which all resources are devoted to growth, and above it to reproduction:

$$\begin{aligned} f_g &= R - f_i \quad a \leqslant w \\ &\quad 0 \qquad\; a > w \\ f_r &= R - f_i \quad a > w. \end{aligned} \tag{4}$$

We assume that the host death rate a particular age, $v(a)$, is determined by two components, namely size, relative to the maximum size at each age, $g_0(a)$, and the current parasite burden, $p(a)$:

$$v(a) = \sigma\left[\left(1 - \frac{g(a)}{g_0(a)}\right) + \beta\, p(a)\right], \tag{5}$$

where β determines the pathogenicity of the parasite ($\beta = 0$ implies that the current parasite burden causes no mortality), and σ is a scaling parameter set to 0·001. Maximum size is calculated from Eqn. 1 with $f_g = R$. The probability of survival of the host to a particular age, $s(a)$, is determined from the differential equation:

$$\frac{ds}{da} = -vs. \tag{6}$$

Relative reproductive output at each age, $m(a)$, is determined as the resources available for reproduction scaled by size (past investment):

$$m(a) = f_r\, g(a). \tag{7}$$

The reproductive value at birth, V, provides a measure of the expected reproductive output at all future ages, weighted by probability of survival to that age:

$$V = \int_0^L m(a)s(a)\, da, \tag{8}$$

where L is the maximum life expectancy and set to 30. This system of equations is solved numerically using standard methods (MatLab, Mathworks Inc).

We are particularly interested in the value of immunity investment, α_{max}, that maximises reproductive value given values of the controlling parameters. The three parameters we consider as controlling are nutritional (resource) input (R), pathogenicity (β) and rate of infection (Λ). We treat these parameters singly, and also consider their interaction, using Monte Carlo simulation to create a community of hosts.

RESULTS

The effect of varying the proportion of resources devoted to immunity (α) and subsequent age-dependent outcomes are illustrated in Fig. 1. These results demonstrate that the reproductive value, V,

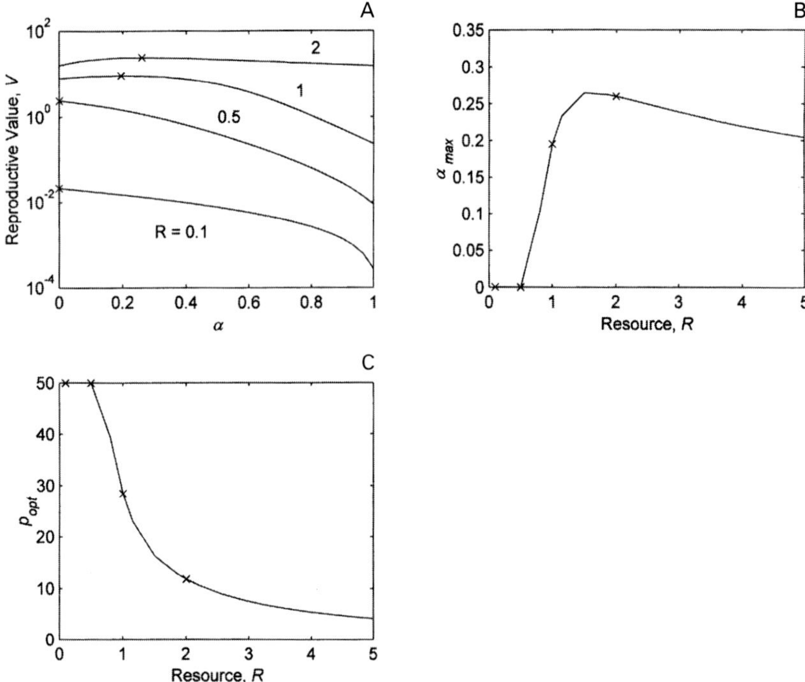

Fig. 2. The relationship between the resource acquisition (R) and maximum immunity resource (α). (a) The reproductive value, V, as a function of α for $R = 0{\cdot}1$, $0{\cdot}5$, 1 and 2 (lines from bottom to top). Note logarithmic scale. The maximum in each case is indicated by x. (b) The value of α that maximises the reproductive value: α_{max}; the points are those in (a). (c) The equilibrium, optimum parasite load (p_{opt}) as a function of R. The points are those in (a) and (b). Other parameters are as Fig. 1.

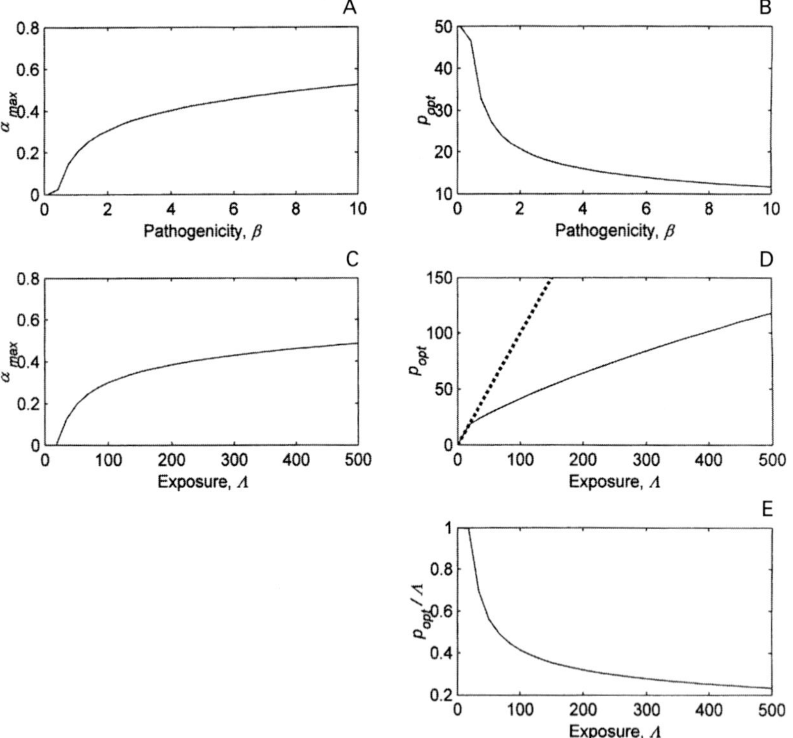

Fig. 3. The relationships between the pathogenicity (β), the rate of infection (Λ) and maximum immunity resource (α). (a) The value of α that maximises the reproductive value, α_{max}, as a function of β. (b) The equilibrium optimum parasite load (p_{opt}) as a function of β. (c) The value of α that maximises the reproductive value, α_{max}, as a function of Λ. (d) The optimum equilibrium parasite load (p_{opt}) as a function of Λ (solid line). The dotted indicates the parasite burden expected with no immunity. (e) As (d), but the parasite burden is plotted as a proportion of the maximum equilibrium, Λ. Other parameters are as Fig. 1.

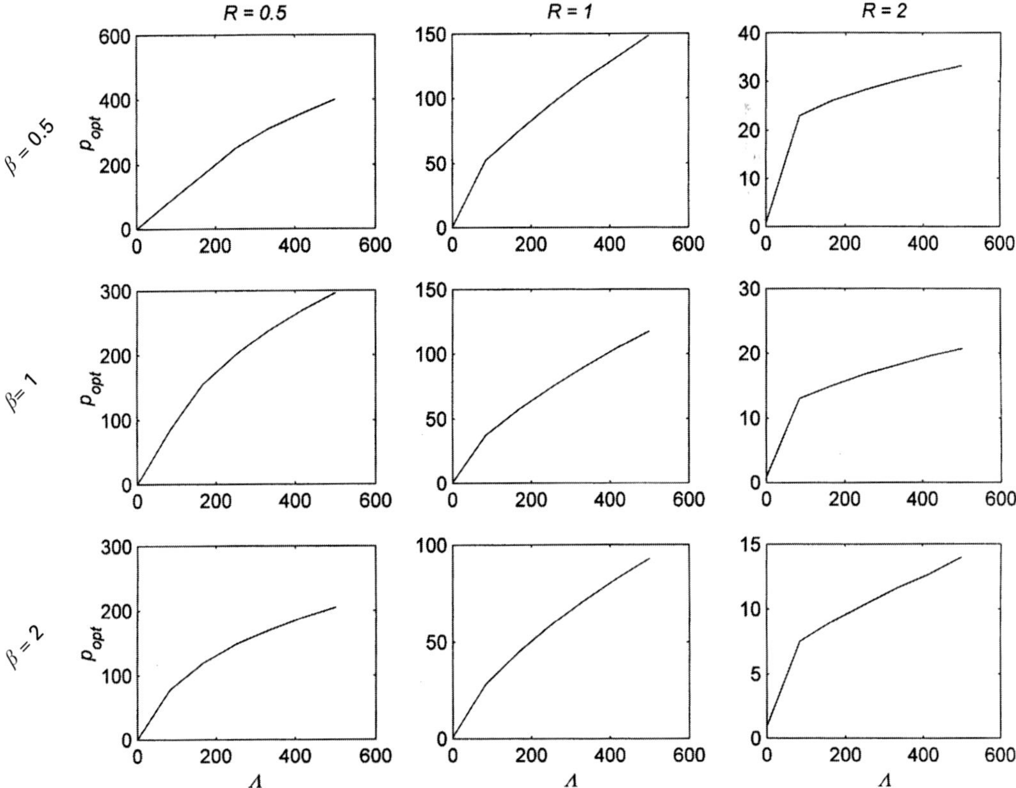

Fig. 4. The interaction between resource acquisition (R), pathogenicity (β) and the rate of infection (Λ). Each graph shows the equilibrium, optimum parasite burden (p_{opt}) as a function of the rate of infection, Λ. The three columns are drawn for $R = 0{\cdot}5$, 1 and 2 (left to right), and the three rows are for $\beta = 0{\cdot}5$, 1 and 2 (top to bottom). Note that the vertical axis is different for each graph.

is maximised when the proportion of resources devoted to immunity is 20% ($\alpha_{max} = 0{\cdot}195$, solid lines). Devoting less (dotted lines) results in a faster growth rate and larger final size (enhancing survival and reproduction) and a higher parasite burden (reducing survival) with a net effect of lower survival. Increasing α (dashed lines) produces a smaller final size (reducing survival and reproduction) and lower parasite burden with consequent higher survival. The reproductive value is, however, lower because of the effect on reproduction, i.e. reproductive output is compromised by using resources to control parasite burden. Note that it is relative values of the reproductive value that are important, rather than absolute value, so that values below unity have no special meaning.

The effect of resource acquisition is demonstrated in Fig. 2. As resource intake is varied, so is the optimal proportion used to control parasite burden. Note that resource acquisition, R, should be interpreted widely, so that it refers not only to direct nutritional uptake, but the host's ability to acquire and utilise resources. Low levels of resource acquisition reduce α_{max}, i.e. the less that is available, the lower the optimum proportion that should be devoted to immunity. At the lowest level shown ($R = 0{\cdot}1$), $\alpha_{max} = 0$ and unrestricted parasite burden is the optimum for the host. Optimal immune allocation increases rapidly for $0{\cdot}5 < R < 1$, and optimal parasite burden falls. For $R > 1{\cdot}5$ the parasite burden can be effectively controlled by reducing the proportion of the (increasing) resources available devoted to immunity.

The effects of variation in pathogenicity, β, and parasite exposure, or infection rate, Λ, are given in Fig. 3. When parasites have no influence on survival (pathogenicity is very low), there is nothing to be gained by controlling them, and the optimum burden is determined by epidemiology alone. As pathogenicity increases so the influence of parasites on survival becomes greater, and the optimum resources devoted to immunity increases (Fig. 3a) and the optimum parasite burden decreases (Fig. 3b). Note again that pathogenicity should be interpreted broadly. It represents the reduction in survival due to parasite infection and will be influenced by both host and parasite factors. Similarly, increasing exposure results in increasing resources devoted to immunity (Fig. 3c). But increasing exposure also increases parasite burden, so that although increasing exposure implies increasing immunity, the net effect remains increasing parasite burden (Fig. 3d, solid line). Consequently, the net effect of immunity is the increasing proportionate reduction of parasite

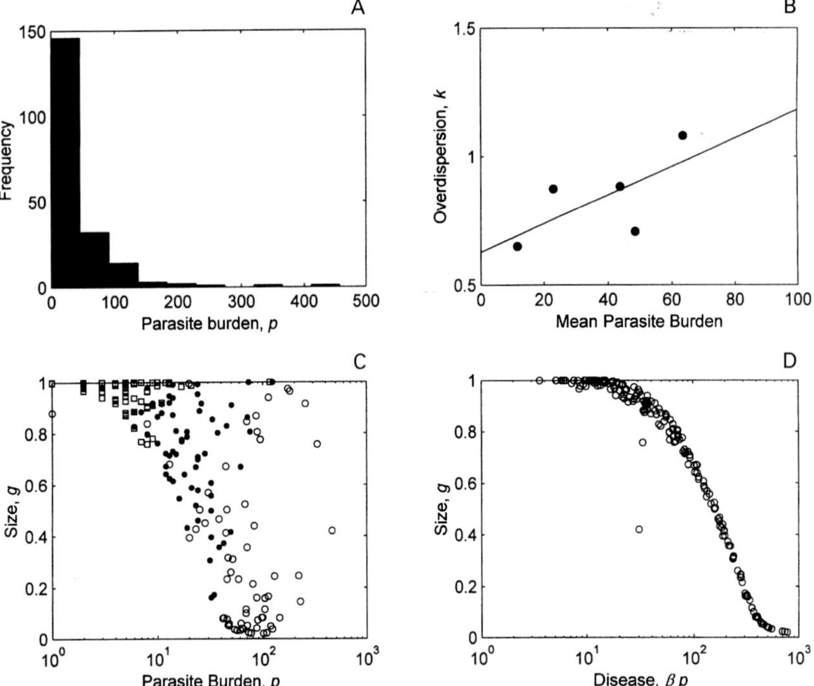

Fig. 5. The distribution and heterogeneity of parasite burdens between 200 different hosts. Each host is assigned a random value for each of three parameters chosen from a uniform distribution: $0{\cdot}4 \leqslant R \leqslant 2{\cdot}4$, $0 \leqslant \Lambda \leqslant 500$ and $0 \leqslant \beta \leqslant 10$. The optimised solution (α_{max}) is found for each individual. The parasite burden and size are taken at age ω. (a) The frequency distribution of the parasite burden. (b) The 200 hosts are divided into 5 equal size groups based on rate of infection, and the mean and overdispersion parameter, k, calculated by maximum likelihood for each group: note k varies inversely with the degree of heterogeneity. The line is found by linear regression. (c) The correlation between size and parasite burden. Note logarithmic axis. The hosts are divided into three equal sized groups based on R: $R < 1{\cdot}1$ (open circles), $1{\cdot}1 < R < 1{\cdot}8$ (closed circles), and $R > 1{\cdot}8$ (open squares). (d) The relationship between size and pathogenic effect of parasite burden (disease). Note logarithmic axis.

burden below the unconstrained value (as measured by the distance between the lines in Fig. 3d drawn in Fig. 3e). These results demonstrate that pathogenicity and exposure are roughly equivalent in terms of optimising the strength of the immune response (compare Fig. 3a with Fig. 3c). The two parameters, Λ and β, are almost linear with regard to the optimisation of host response, apart from the non-linear effect of parasite-induced immune response (eqns 2 and 3). Clearly, either doubling the number of parasites or doubling the effect of a single parasite will have a similar consequence on optimisation of host survival and reproduction. However, increasing Λ results in increase in optimal parasite burdens (from the host's viewpoint), although the proportionate reduction is similar to the effect of pathogenicity (compare Fig. 3b with Fig. 3e).

Fig. 4 shows the effect of simultaneous variation in resource acquisition, pathogenicity and rate of infection in terms of optimum, equilibrium parasite burdens. In all cases, increasing resource acquisition (left to right) results in reduced parasite loads. Increasing pathogenicity (top to bottom) similarly decreases optimum parasite burdens. The optimum parasite burden at extreme rates of infection is relatively little changed by pathogenicity (the effect on survival is already great).

In Fig. 5 we address heterogeneity in parasite burden. These results are simulations of 200 hosts, each of which has a random combination of the parameters R, Λ and β (resource, exposure and pathogenicity respectively). For each host, the optimum parasite burden is calculated and the frequency distribution drawn (Fig. 5a). The result is an overdispersed distribution, mirroring that observed in natural infections, to which a negative binomial distribution provides an empirical description ($k = 0{\cdot}68$). Further, the degree of heterogeneity (as measured inversely by the overdispersion parameter of the negative binomial) appears to decrease as the mean parasite burden increases (Fig. 5b) (although no formal statistics can be calculated).

The relationship between host size, g, and parasite burden, p, is complex (Fig. 5c). Generally, hosts with reduced nutrition (open circles) are smaller but have a wide range of parasite burdens. As resource acquisition increases (filled circles–open squares), size generally increases and parasite burden decreases but there is considerable overlap between these groups. In the low resource group, there is a positive trend in the relationship between size and parasites: larger individuals have a higher burden. As the resource acquisition increases this relationship becomes increasingly negative, so that for the larger individuals, the largest have the smallest burdens.

The total pathogenic effect of infection (or 'disease') is the product of the parasite burden and the pathogenicity of an individual parasite, βp. Since size and disease have the largest impact on reproductive value, the optimisation attempts to find the most profitable relationship between these two variables (Fig. 5d). This relationship is not causal: it represents the optimum an individual can achieve given the circumstances. So that, remembering that size is a proxy measure for condition or investment for future reproduction and survival, it would be erroneous to conclude, for example, that disease causes small size.

DISCUSSION

This is, to the best of my knowledge, the first quantitative description of the immunological and epidemiological effects of resource partitioning between immunity, growth and reproduction from an individual host perspective. The first conclusion is that hosts' attempts to maximise their resource use under conditions of continuous infection will generally result in co-existence with parasite infection. 'Failure' to control parasites does not mean immunological failure or parasite evasion of immunity – a non-zero parasite burden can be an optimal strategy for the host (Fig. 1) (Behnke *et al.* 1992).

Variation in resource acquisition results in a change in this parasite burden (Fig. 2). With this model and parameters, the effect of resource acquisition on parasite burdens is highly non-linear and produces a threshold effect – malnourished hosts have high burdens and little immunity, well nourished hosts have low burdens, and there is a switch between the two over a short range of R. Perhaps of greatest significance is that individuals on very low nutritional planes should put increasingly less resources into immunity. This would be further extenuated if resource acquisition was positively related to size, or inversely related to parasite burden. In this case, even small initial differences might have very large consequences. Resource acquisition is highly predictive of reproductive value. Fig. 3 demonstrates that although optimisation in the face of varying pathogenicity and rate of infection have similar immunological effects, they have very different epidemiological consequences, i.e. opposite effects on absolute parasite burden.

The epidemiological (population) consequences of hosts specific optimisation are interesting. Each host will have a different optimal response, largely because they have different resources bases, and different 'views' of the parasite (e.g. what is pathogenic to one host might be benign to another), and will be exposed to different numbers of different parasite strains. These differences will be multi-dimensional and include genetic, environmental and chance components. The results suggestion that we can interpret heterogeneity in parasite burden in terms of individual hosts finding their own optimum immune response, and therefore their own optimum parasite burden. Changes in the epidemiology of infection can result in 'shuffling' of the hosts' parasite burdens, rather than necessarily changing the mean parasite burden. Consequently, continued exposure might be expected to have as great an effect on the variability of parasite burden between hosts as on average burdens. The observation that individual hosts are predisposed to relative parasite burdens is consistent with this view – individuals' optima are relatively constant within a group of hosts. Epidemiological investigations frequently involve comparisons between communities. However, it is within the individual host that infection and immunity occur, so that community or population level phenomena are the manifestation of processes and effects operating within individual hosts. The framework presented here has potential for investigating the community-level manifestations of individual host processes. When variation in controlling parameters (resource acquisition, exposure and pathogenicity) is included, the distribution of parasite burdens (each being the host's own, personal optimum) is overdispersed (Fig. 5). In principle this is because the combination of conditions that optimise a high burden is relatively rare. Further, the variation takes the same form as that observed – i.e. it decreases as the mean increases. In field data, the relationship between parasite burden and condition (e.g. size) is frequently difficult to demonstrate. As each host is optimising its own circumstances to reduce the impact of parasites, this impact can be unclear from observational data. In well-nourished individuals, this relationship may be positive, i.e. hosts in better condition have more parasites.

The model presented is clearly simplified in many respects. In particular, physiology, immunity, life history and parasite infection present a complex, non-linear interaction of processes that have not been fully addressed. For example, the age of sexual maturity (w) should itself be dependent on size (g), and size may have a non-linear effect on reproductive success (Hurd, 2001) and resource acquisition. Further, we only consider host adaptation to parasite infection. Parasites themselves are subject *inter alia* to the trade-off between transmission and reduced survival in hosts, considerably complicating the interaction (van Baalen, 1998; Hurd, 2001). One of the major hurdles to overcome in experimental testing of hypotheses is the nature of this interaction. For example, pathology (= reduced survival) must be viewed in an evolutionary context, which is itself the context for epidemiology and hence pathology. Competition experiments have proved useful in evolutionary (i.e. strictly genetic) investigations (e.g. Kraaijeveld & Godfray, 1997), but demonstrating that hosts have obtained a constrained optimum within their lifetime is potentially more difficult to confirm experimentally.

The immune response to infection is complicated. In part, this complexity in mechanism derives from complexity in function, which is not only to control infection and disease, but to do so in the most cost-effective manner. For example, the commitment to Th1 or Th2 response should be viewed not only in terms of its effect on host protection (Jankovic, Liu & Gause, 2001), but also its consequent effect on physiology, its physiological cost and other aspects of immunity (Yazdanbakhsh, van den Biggelaar & Maizels, 2001; Matarese *et al.* 2002). Another complication is that multiple parasite infections of a single host are the norm (Graham, 2001). Not surprisingly, there is substantial evidence for a close interaction between immunity and physiology (for example of the interaction between immunity and CNS, see Anisman, Zalcman & Zacharko, 1993), as well as environmentally mediated effects (e.g. Nelson & Demas, 1996). Our results do not depend on the immune response being able to distinguish protective from non-protective responses. A parasite that is able to subvert host immune resources to non-protective antigens (which reduces the immune effectiveness) will presumably increase the optimum burden (from the hosts' viewpoint). This could be included in the model in eqn 3 (which implicitly assumes that all resources devoted to immunity have a linear impact on parasite establishment). The outcome here is related to the resources devoted to immunity and it would clearly be in the host's interest to ensure that these resources are used effectively. In addition to the direct costs of mounting an immune response, most such responses result in some form of immunopathology (Garside *et al.* 2000), where again hosts are having to compromise between killing parasites and self-damage as a consequence. Model simulations including immunopathology (by making survival dependent on both immune function and parasites in eqn 5) do indeed suggest that optimum investment in immunity is reduced and parasite burden increased (results not shown).

Throughout, we have only considered a constant (lifetime) investment in immunity. However, hosts are likely to adjust apportionment of resources in real time, i.e. optimising at each age (though the returns are determined over the host's lifetime). Age-related strategies will be a result of both host optimisation and age-related exposure. Environmental influences (including infection) during early life can have pervasive effects at later ages (e.g. Metcalfe & Monaghan, 2001). Consequently, the immunological response will be highly age-dependent, and will greatly influence the age-related epidemiology of pathogens. Likewise, 'immaturity' of the immune response in young individuals may be shown to be an adaptive approach to resource allocation: an optimum strategy might be to permit higher parasite burdens (and risk morbidity and mortality) in return for being in a better state to reproduce later. Hosts might be expected to differentiate between infecting parasites (in terms of, say, pathogenicity) in determining the level of immune response to each. For example, it would make evolutionary sense to react quickly to a multiplying virus that would kill if uncontrolled which, given constraints, will likely imply reduction of immunity directed against parasites that are less dangerous. This requires mechanisms (within the immune system) that are capable of detecting changes in abundance and spatial distribution of parasites within the host, and determining morbid consequences of each parasite population. Suppression of subsets of the immune response through activation of others need not be directly due to the parasites themselves but an effect of host resource allocation (Moret & Schmid-Hempel, 2000). Consequently, elimination of one pathogen may enhance the immune response to others (Bundy, Sher & Michael, 2000).

One consequence of acknowledging that hosts must optimise resource allocation is that individual hosts have to find their own optimal parasite burden. Depending on the speed with which this optimisation occurs, this would result in changes in the distribution of parasite burdens with age, which would also be exacerbated by changes in the optimum with age (Pacala & Dobson, 1988). Aspects of the immune system are transferred from mother to offspring (Carlier & Truyens, 1995). Could not mechanisms exist to pass information about, say, the pathogenicity of specific infections? The neonate that received 'immunological wisdom' from its mother would be in a much better position to juggle resource allocation between growth and immunity than one that was ignorant. Such direct maternal effects will confound analyses based solely on the assumption of genetic transfer of information.

In summary, the general, quantitative framework presented is a step towards further understanding of the interaction between immunity and epidemiology. The model makes the undesirable assumption that the immune system is optimising in order to understand the potential epidemiological consequences (Parker & Maynard Smith, 1990). It is to be hoped that future work will develop better understanding of the constraints and context within which the immune system functions.

ACKNOWLEDGEMENTS

I thank Jaap Boes, Shana Coates, Peter Nansen, Jan Roger and Lisa White and for useful discussions and comments.

REFERENCES

ANDERSON, R. M. & MEDLEY, G. F. (1985). Community control of helminth infections of man by mass and selective chemotherapy. *Parasitology* **90**, 629–660.

ANISMAN, H., ZALCMAN, S. & ZACHARKO, R. M. (1993). The impact of stressors on immune and central neurotransmitter activity: bidirectional communication. *Reviews in the Neurosciences* **4**, 147–180.

ANTONOVICS, J. & THRALL, P. H. (1994). The cost of resistance and the maintenance of genetic polymorphism in the host-pathogen systems. *Proceedings of the Royal Society of London, Series B* **257**, 105–110.

BARNARD, C. J., BEHNKE, J. M., GAGE, A. R., BROWN, H. & SMITHURST, P. R. (1997). Immunity costs and behavioural modulation in male laboratory mice (*Mus musculus*) exposed to the odours of females. *Physiology and Behavior* **62**, 857–866.

BEHNKE, J. M., BARNARD, C. J. & WAKELIN, D. (1992). Understanding chronic nematode infections: evolutionary considerations, current hypotheses and the way forward. *International Journal for Parasitology* **22**, 861–907.

BOES, J., COATES, S., MEDLEY, G. F., VARADY, M., ERIKSEN, L., ROEPSTORFF, A. & NANSEN, P. (1999). The role of material immunity in experimental *Ascaris suum* infections in young piglets. *Parasitology* **119**, 509–520.

BOES, J., MEDLEY, G. F., ERIKSEN, L., ROEPSTORFF, A. & NANSEN, P. (1998). Distribution of *Ascaris suum* in experimentally and naturally infected pigs and comparison with *Ascaris lumbricoides* infections in humans. *Parasitology* **117**, 589–596.

BOOTS, M. & BEGON, M. (1993). Trade-offs with resistance to a granulosis virus in the Indian meal moth, examined by a laboratory evolution experiment. *Functional Ecology* **7**, 528–534.

BOWERS, R. G., BOOTS, M. & BEGON, M. (1994). Life-history trade-offs and the evolution of pathogen resistance: competition between host strains. *Proceedings of the Royal Society of London, Series B* **257**, 247–253.

BUNDY, D. A. P. & MEDLEY, G. F. (1992). Immuno-epidemiology of human geohelminthiasis: ecological and immunological determinants of worm burden. *Parasitology* **104**, S105–S119.

BUNDY, D. A. P., SHER, A. & MICHAEL, E. (2000). Good worms or bad worms: do worm infections affect the epidemiological patterns of other diseases? *Parasitology Today* **16**, 273–274.

CARLIER, Y. & TRUYENS, C. (1995). Influence of maternal infection on offspring resistance towards parasites. *Parasitology Today* **11**, 94–99.

CHAN, L., BUNDY, D. A. P. & KAN, S. P. (1994*a*). Aggregation and predisposition to *Ascaris lumbricoides* and *Trichuris trichiura* at the familial level. *Transactions of the Royal Society of Tropical Medicine and Hygiene* **88**, 46–48.

CHAN, L., BUNDY, D. A. P. & KAN, S. P. (1994*b*). Genetic relatedness as a determinant of predisposition to *Ascaris lumbricoides* and *Trichuris trichiura* infection. *Parasitology* **108**, 77–80.

COOP, R. L. & KYRIAZAKIS, I. (1999). Nutrition-parasite interaction. *Veterinary Parasitology* **84**, 187–204.

FELLOWES, M. D. E., KRAAIJEVELD, A. R. & GODFRAY, H. C. J. (1998). Trade-off associated with selection for increased ability to resist parasitoid attack in *Drosophila melanogaster*. *Proceedings of the Royal Society of London, Series B* **265**, 1553–1558.

GARSIDE, P., KENNEDY, M. W., WAKELIN, D. & LAWRENCE, C. E. (2000). Immunopathology of intestinal helminth infection. *Parasite Immunology* **22**, 605–612.

GRAHAM, A. L. (2001). Use of an optimality model to solve the immunological puzzle of concomitant infection. *Parasitology* **122**, S61–S64.

GUSTAFSSON, L., NORDLING, D., ANDERSSON, M. S., SHELDON, B. C. & QVARNSTROM, A. (1994). Infectious diseases, reproductive effort and the cost of reproduction in birds. *Philosophical Transactions of the Royal Society of London, Series B* **346**, 323–331.

GUYATT, H. L., BUNDY, D. A. P., MEDLEY, G. F. & GRENFELL, B. T. (1990). The relationship between the frequency distribution of *Ascaris lumbricoides* and the prevalence and intensity of infection in human communities. *Parasitology* **101**, 139–143.

GUYATT, H. L., SMITH, T., GRYSEELS, B., LENGELER, C., MSHINDA, H., SIZIYA, S., SALANAVE, B., MOHOME, N., MAKWALA, J., NGIMBI, K. P. & TANNER, M. (1994). Aggregation in schistosomiasis: comparison of the relationships between prevalence and intensity in different endemic areas. *Parasitology* **109**, 45–55.

HUDSON, P. J. & DOBSON, A. P. (1995). Macroparasites: observed patterns in naturally fluctuating animal populations. In *Ecology of Infectious Diseases in Natural Populations* (ed. Grenfell, B. T. & Dobson, A. P.). Cambridge, Cambridge University Press.

HURD, H. (2001). Host fecundity reduction: a strategy for damage limitation? *Trends in Parasitology* **17**, 363–368.

JANKOVIC, D., LIU, Z. & GAUSE, W. C. (2001). Th1- and Th2-cell commitment during infectious disease: asymmetry in divergent pathways. *Trends in Immunology* **22**, 450–457.

KAITALA, V., HEINO, M. & GETZ, W. M. (1997). Host-parasite dynamics and the evolution of host immunity and parasite fecundity strategies. *Bulletin of Mathematical Biology* **59**, 427–450.

KEYMER, A. E. & PAGEL, M. (1990). Predisposition to hookworm infection. In *Hookworm Infection: Current Status and New Directions* (ed. Schad, G. A. & Warren, K. S.). London, Taylor and Francis.

KRAAIJEVELD, A. R. & GODFRAY, H. C. J. (1997). Trade-off between parasitoid resistance and larval competitive ability in *Drosophila melanogaster*. *Nature* **389**, 278–280.

LOCHMILLER, R. L. & DEERENBERG, C. (2000). Trade-offs in evolutionary immunology: just what are the costs of immunity? *Oikos* **88**, 87–98.

LWAMBO, N. J. S., BUNDY, D. A. P. & MEDLEY, G. F. H. (1992). A new approach to morbidity risk assessment in hookworm endemic communities. *Epidemiology and Infection* **108**, 469–481.

MATARESE, G., LA CAVA, A., SANNA, V., LORD, G. M., LECHLER, R. I., FONTANA, S. & ZAPPACOSTA, S. (2002). Balancing susceptibility to infection and autoimmunity: a role for leptin? *Trends in Immunology* **23**, 182–187.

MEDLEY, G. F. & BUNDY, D. A. P. (1996). Dynamic modelling of epidemiological patterns of schistosomiasis morbidity. *American Journal of Tropical Medicine and Hygiene* **55**, 149–158.

MEDLEY, G. F., SINDEN, R. E., FLECK, S., BILLINGSLEY, P. F., TIRAWANCHAI, N. & RODRIGUEZ, M. H. (1993). Heterogeneity in patterns of malarial oocyst infections in the mosquito vector. *Parasitology* **106**, 441–449.

METCALFE, N. B. & MONAHAN, P. (2001). Compensation of a bad start: grow now, pay later? *Trends in Ecology and Evolution* **16**, 254–260.

MICHAEL, E. & BUNDY, D. A. P. (1992*a*). Nutrition, immunity and helminth infection: effects of dietary protein in the dynamics of the primary antibody response to *Trichuris muris* (Nematoda) in CBA/Ca mice. *Parasite Immunology* **14**, 169–183.

MICHAEL, E. & BUNDY, D. A. P. (1992*b*). Protein content of CBA/Ca mouse diet: relationship with host antibody responses and the population dynamics of *Trichuris muris* (Nematoda) in repeated infection. *Parasitology* **105**, 139–150.

MORET, Y. & SCHMID-HEMPEL, P. (2000). Survival for immunity: the price of immune system activation for bumblebee workers. *Science* **290**, 1166–1168.

NELSON, R. J. & DEMAS, G. E. (1996). Seasonal changes in immune function. *The Quarterly Review of Biology* **71**, 511–548.

PACALA, S. W. & DOBSON, A. P. (1988). The relation between the number of parasites/host and host age: population dynamic causes and maximum likelihood estimation. *Parasitology* **96**, 197–210.

PARKER, G. A. & MAYNARD SMITH, J. (1990). Optimality theory in evolutionary biology. *Nature* **348**, 27–33.

PETKEVICIUS, S., BJORN, H., ROEPSTORFF, A., NANSEN, P., BACH KNUDSEN, K. E., BARNES, E. H. & JENSEN, K. (1995). The effect of two types of diet on populations of *Ascaris suum* and *Oesophagostomum dentatum* in experimentally infected pigs. *Parasitology* **111**, 395–402.

QUINNELL, R. J., MEDLEY, G. F. & KEYMER, A. E. (1990). The regulation of gastro-intestinal helminth populations. *Proceedings of the Royal Society of London, Series B* **330**, 191–201.

READ, A. F. & ALLEN, E. A. (2000). The economics of immunity. *Science* **290**, 1104–1105.

ROEPSTORFF, A., ERIKSEN, L., SLOTVED, H. C. & NANSEN, P. (1997). Experimental *Ascaris suum* infection in the pig: worm population kinetics following single inoculations with three doses of infective eggs. *Parasitology* **115**, 443–452.

SHELDON, B. C. & VERHULST, S. (1996). Ecological immunology: costly parasite defences and trade-offs in evolutionary ecology. *Trends in Ecology and Evolution* **11**, 317–321.

VAN BAALEN, M. (1998). Coevolution of recovery ability and virulence. *Proceedings of the Royal Society of London, Series B* **265**, 317–325.

WILLIAMS-BLANGERO, S., SUBEDI, J., UPADHAYAY, R. P., MANRAL, D. B., RAI, D. R., JHA, B., ROBINSON, E. S. & BLANGERO, J. (1999). Genetic analysis of susceptibility to infection with *Ascaris lumbricoides*. *American Journal of Tropical Medicine & Hygiene* **60**, 921–926.

WOOLHOUSE, M. E. J. (1992). A theoretical framework for the immunoepidemiology of helminth infection. *Parasite Immunology* **14**, 563–578.

YAZDANBAKHSH, M., VAN DEN BIGGELAAR, A. & MAIZELS, R. M. (2001). Th2 responses without atopy: immunoregulation in chronic helminth infections and reduced allergic disease. *Trends in Immunology* **22**, 372–377.

Costs of resistance in insect-parasite and insect-parasitoid interactions

A. R. KRAAIJEVELD*, J. FERRARI *and* H. C. J. GODFRAY

NERC Centre for Population Biology and Department of Biological Sciences, Imperial College at Silwood Park, Ascot, Berks, SL5 7PY, UK

SUMMARY

Most, if not all, organisms face attack by natural enemies and will be selected to evolve some form of defence. Resistance may have costs as well as its obvious benefits. These costs may be associated with actual defence or with the maintenance of the defensive machinery irrespective of whether a challenge occurs. In this paper, the evidence for costs of resistance in insect-parasite and insect-parasitoid systems is reviewed, with emphasis on two host-parasitoid systems, based on *Drosophila melanogaster* and pea aphids as hosts. Data from true insect-parasite systems mainly concern the costs of actual defence; evidence for the costs of standing defences is mostly circumstantial. In pea aphids, the costs of standing defences have so far proved elusive. Resistance amongst clones is not correlated with life-time fecundity, whether measured on good or poor quality plants. Successful defence by a *D. melanogaster* larva results in a reduction in adult size and fecundity and an increased susceptibility to pupal parasitoids. Costs of standing defences are a reduction in larval competitive ability though these costs only become important when food is limited. It is concluded that costs of resistance can play a pivotal role in the evolutionary and population dynamic interactions between hosts and their parasites.

Key words: Costs of resistance, host, immunity, parasite, parasitoid, trade-off.

INTRODUCTION

Almost all organisms face attack by predators and parasites and will therefore be selected to evolve some sort of defence mechanism against these natural enemies. Especially in the last decade, it has become increasingly clear that resistance against pathogens and parasites can be a mixed blessing, as high levels of resistance have their costs. Costs of resistance to natural enemies have been identified in organisms as varied as *Escherichia coli* (Lenski, 1988), plants (Bergelson & Purrington, 1996), snails (Webster & Woolhouse, 1999; Rigby & Jokela, 2000) and birds (Sheldon & Verhulst, 1996; Verhulst, Dieleman & Parmentier, 1999). The rate and direction of the evolution of resistance will depend on the combination of the selection pressures exerted by natural enemies and the nature and magnitude of the costs of resistance.

It is important to distinguish between two types of costs of resistance. First, the costs of *actual defence*, which are borne after an individual is parasitised. These costs arise as a result of energy and other resources being used in the deployment of the immune system (and/or other defences) following parasitism. The other type of cost is that of *standing defences*. This type of cost is associated with investment in the immune system (or any other defence mechanism) in anticipation of potential future parasitism.

* Author for correspondence: A. R. Kraaijeveld. Tel: +44-20-75942544; Fax: +44-1344-873173. E-mail: a.kraayeveld@ic.ac.uk

Costs of actual defence will influence the evolution of resistance. When successful defence has negative effects on other fitness parameters, the spread of resistance genes in a population will be slowed down. If costs are so high that parasitised individuals that have successfully defended themselves against the parasite do not leave any offspring, resistance cannot evolve at all. Resistance will also not evolve if the costs of actual defence are greater than the negative effect the parasite has on the host. The costs of standing defences can also influence whether resistance will evolve: if costs of standing defence are high and the probability of being parasitised is low, there will be selection for low levels or the absence of resistance. In a system in which the natural enemy obligatorily prevents its host from producing any offspring, costs of standing defence are the only type of costs that will influence the evolution of resistance.

We first give an overview of insect-parasite systems where costs, or indications of costs, have been found. Then we review in more detail our present state of knowledge of two well-studied insect-parasitoid systems, based on pea aphids and *Drosophila melanogaster* as hosts. Because parasitoids always kill their host, selection pressures on defence and counter-defence in host-parasitoid interactions are often stronger than in typical host-parasite systems.

Costs of actual defence

The clearest example that the employment of the immune system is costly comes from bumble bees (*Bombus terrestris*). Starved and non-starved bees

Parasitology (2002), **125**, S71–S82. © 2002 Cambridge University Press
DOI: 10.1017/S0031182002001750 Printed in the United Kingdom

were challenged with either lipopolysaccharides extracted from *Escherichia coli* or bacteria-sized latex beads. Lipopolysaccharides are cell-surface molecules used by the immune system to recognise bacteria; the reason behind injecting these or the latex beads was to challenge the immune system with substances that have no pathogenic effect *per se*. In the starved bees, the induction of the immune system led to a reduction in survival compared to non-starved bees (Moret & Schmid-Hempel, 2000). Limiting the resource uptake by starving the bees reveals that employing the immune system has costs. These costs remain hidden in bees that have abundant food and therefore do not need to partition limited resources between the immune system and somatic maintenance.

Often it is difficult to distinguish costs of actual defence from the negative effects of the parasite. Mosquitoes (*Armigerus subalbatus*) which have encapsulated filarial worms show reduced and delayed egg-laying (Ferdig *et al.* 1993), but it is unclear whether this is a cost of the encapsulation process itself or a pathogenic effect of the parasites, or even a combination of both. Bumble bee colonies, in which the workers received an immune challenge with lipopolysaccharides, had lower overall reproductive output and produced fewer queens (Moret & Schmid-Hempel, 2001). As lipopolysaccharides have no pathogenic effect themselves, this suggests a trade-off between actual defence and reproduction on a colony level.

A direct indication that resources involved in mounting an immune response are limiting within an individual comes from the damselfly, *Mnais costalis*. Phenoloxidase is a key enzyme in the immune system of many insects (Nappi, 1975; Lackie, 1988*a*). Siva-Jothy *et al.* (2001) injected nylon filaments into the haemolymph of field-caught adult damselflies. In individuals which received such an acute immune challenge, there was a negative correlation between phenoloxidase activity and eugregarine parasite burden in the midgut. No such correlation was found in individuals that did not receive an acute immune challenge. This suggests that maintaining high phenoloxidase levels in both parts of the organism (the haemolymph and the midgut) is costly. Bumble bee workers which have been challenged with lipopolysaccharides (which, as explained above, have no pathogenic effects themselves) show an increased antibacterial activity but a reduction in phenoloxidase activity (Moret & Schmid-Hempel, 2001). This is an indication of a trade-off between the two different immune responses.

Further indications that resisting parasites is costly come from observations that levels of immunity are reduced when the animal is concentrating resources in other activities. For instance, an increase in reproductive activity is correlated with a reduction in levels of defence, as measured by the immune response against an injected nylon filament in males and females of the damselfly, *Matrona basilaris japonica*, (Siva-Jothy, Tsubaki & Hooper, 1998) and against bacteria in *D. melanogaster* males (McKean & Nunney, 2001). An increase in foraging activity is correlated with a reduction in the immune response against an injected nylon filament in bumble bees (König & Schmid-Hempel, 1995; Doums & Schmid-Hempel, 2000).

Indication of a very different kind, that up-regulation of the immune system can be costly, comes from a genome-wide analysis (using oligonucleotide microarrays) of the immune response of *D. melanogaster* against infection with bacteria and entomopathogenic fungi (De Gregorio *et al.* 2001). *Drosophila melanogaster* adults which received a septic injury with a needle dipped in a culture of *E. coli* and *Micrococcus luteus*, or were infected with *Beauvaria bassiana*, showed increased expression of 230 genes. A discussion of these genes, and their role in the immune reaction, is beyond the scope of this paper, but the authors also found 170 genes which were down-regulated. Among these were genes that are involved in general metabolism. It is possible that the up-regulation of the many genes involved in the immune reaction, and the resources involved, requires a down-regulation of metabolic processes which are not immediately necessary, with potential consequences for other fitness parameters.

Costs of standing defences

The most powerful methods to identify trade-offs between resistance and other fitness parameters are quantitative genetic estimation of trait covariance and selection experiments (Reznick, 1985). Apart from the examples mentioned in the next section, very few data using one of these methodologies exist in the literature. Evolution of resistance against a granulosis virus is correlated with longer developmental time and reduction in egg viability in the Indian meal moth (*Plodia interpunctella*; Boots & Begon, 1993). A mosquito (*Aedes aegypti*) line resistant to the malaria parasite had smaller adult body size, lower fecundity and shorter longevity than a susceptible line (Yan, Severson & Christensen, 1997). A problem with both these studies, however, is a lack of replication across lines.

Phenotypic correlations between resistance and other traits can provide circumstantial evidence that resistance is costly, but the possibility that there is an unknown third variable underlying the correlation cannot be ruled out. Nevertheless, the results of a number of studies are consistent with resources being required for maintenance of a high level of standing defence.

Several insect species show phenotypic plasticity in a range of traits depending on population density. The best example of this 'density-dependent phase polyphenism' are desert locusts, *Schistocerca gregaria* (Pener & Yerushalmi, 1998). High-density forms are often darker and a potential explanation is that the cuticle is heavily melanised and hardened to resist parasite attack, which is more likely to occur in high density populations. Darker (gregarious) forms of *Spodoptera* spp. and *Tenebrio molitor* are indeed more resistant to pathogens and parasitoids (Reeson *et al.* 1998; Barnes & Siva-Jothy, 2000; Wilson *et al.* 2001). Phenoloxidase levels are also increased in gregarious forms (Reeson *et al.* 1998; Wilson *et al.* 2001). This again may be due to higher risks of infection. However, if cuticular melanisation had evolved for another reason, for example thermo-regulation, and if cuticle hardening and the immune system shared metabolic pathways, as appears to be the case, then the marginal costs of maintaining high levels of immune function may be lower in gregarious forms and thus greater activity might be selected in the absence of a difference in risk of infection. Interestingly, when bumble bee workers were immunologically challenged by lipopolysaccharides, the males produced by these colonies show an increase in phenoloxidase activity (Moret & Schmid-Hempel, 2001). The physiological mechanism of this trans-generation transfer of increased immunity is unknown, but conceptually it is similar to what may be happening in phase-dependent polyphenic insects: costly up-regulation of the immune system only when there is an indication for an increased risk of infection.

Gender differences in investment in immune function are found in a handful of insect species (Kurtz *et al.* 2000 and references therein). In general, males have a lower level of immune function than females, which appears to result from a trade-off between investment in resistance and in sexual traits and activity. In several insect species, females prefer males exhibiting indications of higher immune function. Males of the damselfly, *Calopteryx splendens xanthostoma*, with darker wing spots are preferred by females and have higher resistance against eugregarine parasites (Siva-Jothy, 2000). Phenoloxidase is involved in the deposition of melanin in the wings (Siva-Jothy, 2000). It is hypothesised that individuals with a strong immune system are better able to provide dark wing spots (a revealing handicap) or that high quality males can afford to invest in both wing pigmentation and defence. Cricket (*Acheta domesticus*) females prefer males with more syllables per chirp in their song. There is a positive correlation between number of syllables per chirp and both haemocyte numbers and encapsulation ability in males (Ryder & Siva-Jothy, 2000).

COSTS OF RESISTANCE TO PARASITOIDS

Parasitoids are intermediate between true parasites and predators in that they are parasitic in their host as larvae, but at some point in their development kill their host and become free-living adults (Godfray, 1994). Because only one of the two combatants can survive parasitism, there is strong selection on hosts to be resistant, and on parasitoids to evolve counter-defence mechanisms. Unlike the case with true parasites, where the costs of actual defence may be greater than the harmful effect of the parasite, the costs of actual defence against parasitoids with always have to be paid, as the alternative for the host is death.

Apart from the two insect-parasitoid systems that we discuss below, there is little evidence on the nature and magnitude of the costs of resistance against parasitoids (the older literature is reviewed by Godfray, 1994, and Kraaijeveld, van Alphen & Godfray, 1998). In the pyralid, *Corcyra cephalonica*, attacked by the ichneumonid, *Venturia canescens*, the development time of surviving moths increases the more parasitoid eggs are encapsulated by the larva (Harvey, Thompson & Heyes, 1996). This may indeed be a cost of actual defence, but it is difficult to separate the effects of employing the immune system from the direct harm done to the host by the ovipositing parasitoid. Work by Zareh, Westoby & Pimentel (1980) hints at costs of standing defences in house flies (*Musca domestica*) against the pupal parasitoid, *Nasonia vitripennis*. Fly lines exposed to parasitism evolved heavier puparia and a shorter pupal stage duration. Presumably these trait changes are adaptations to reduce the risk of parasitism and can therefore be seen as resistance mechanisms. Zareh *et al.* (1980) found a reduction in female fecundity in the lines exposed to parasitoids, possibly a direct effect of the shorter pupal stage.

Pea aphids

Pea aphids (*Acyrthosiphon pisum*, Homoptera, Aphididae) are cyclical parthenogens that feed on a range of legume species. The two most common parasitoid species that attack pea aphids are the braconids, *Aphidius ervi* and *A. eadyi*. The former also attacks a number of related aphid species, while *A. eadyi* is a specialist on pea aphids (Starý, González & Hall, 1980; Müller *et al.* 1999). In addition, pea aphids are subject to infection by a number of fungi, of which *Erynia neoaphidis* (Entomophthorales, Entomophthoraceae) is the most common, at least in southern England.

How pea aphids defend themselves against parasitoids and fungi is unknown. What is clear, however, is that encapsulation, the prime cellular defence mechanism in insects, plays no role (Milner, 1982; Henter & Via, 1995). At single sites, there is

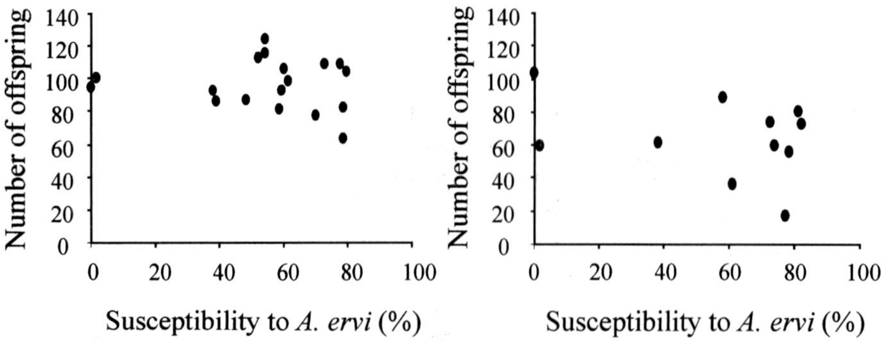

Fig. 1. Correlation amongst *Acyrthosiphon pisum* clones between susceptibility to *Aphidius ervi* and offspring production on (a) good and (b) poor quality host plants. See Ferrari *et al.* (2001) for experimental details.

substantial between-clone variation in resistance against *A. ervi*, *A. eadyi* and *E. neoaphidis* (Henter & Via, 1995; Ferrari *et al.* 2001). Among populations, the picture is complicated by the host plant specialisation of pea aphids. The species feeds on a wide range of legume species, but individual genotypes are very specialised on different plant species (Via, 1991 *a*, *b*, 1999; Sandström, 1994; Sandström & Petterson, 1994; Via, Bouck & Skillman, 2000). In two separate areas of the United States, pea aphids specialised on *Medicago sativa* were more resistant to *A. ervi* than aphids from *Trifolium pratense* (Hufbauer & Via, 1999; Hufbauer, 2001).

Within one field of *M. sativa*, Henter & Via (1995) did not observe an increase in the frequency of resistant clones in a population over the course of a field season despite variation in resistance among clones and substantial rates of parasitism. One explanation for this is that costs of resistance are important. So far, however, the nature and magnitude of the costs of resistance in pea aphids has proved elusive. We measured the resistance of over 28 pea aphid clones to *A. ervi*, *A. eadyi* and *E. neoaphidis* and, for a subset of clones, life-time fecundity on good and poor quality plants (Ferrari *et al.* 2001). No correlation across clones between resistance to any of the three natural enemies and life-time fecundity was found (Fig. 1 shows the results for *A. ervi*).

Across clones, resistance against *A. ervi* and *A. eadyi* is positively correlated (Ferrari *et al.* 2001). Some clones are almost completely susceptible to both species, while others are completely resistant. However, several clones are more resistant to the specialist *A. eadyi* than to the generalist *A. ervi* (Fig. 2*a*). These results were complicated by the observation that some clones which survived attack by *A. eadyi* (our definition of resistance) produced virtually no offspring after successful defence. Parasites and parasitoids often shut down host investment in reproduction which is wasteful from the parasite's point of view. This may be why some of the clones produced no offspring, even though they did defend themselves successfully against the parasitoid. Cross-resistance between parasitoids and the fungus, *E. neoaphidis*, is not significantly correlated, though there is a positive trend (Fig. 2*b*; Ferrari *et al.* 2001).

We have limited evidence that the relative resistance of different aphid clones remains the same when challenged by different parasitoid genotypes. Resistance of British pea aphid clones to a British strain of *A. ervi* was highly and positively correlated with resistance against an American strain (unpublished data). Furthermore, there is no evidence that parasitoids collected on different host plant species survived better on aphids from their own host plant species compared with aphids from other host plant species (Hufbauer, 2001).

Drosophila melanogaster

D. melanogaster is among the more common *Drosophila* species breeding in fermenting fruits. Its larvae are attacked by several parasitoid species, of which the most common in Europe are the braconid, *Asobara tabida*, and the figitids, *Leptopilina heterotoma* and *L. boulardi* (Carton *et al.* 1986). Like many insects and other invertebrates (Nappi, 1975; Lackie, 1988 *a*, *b*), *D. melanogaster* larvae are able to mount a cellular immune response, called encapsulation, against parasitism (Nappi, 1975; Rizki & Rizki, 1984; Strand & Pech, 1995). First, the parasitoid egg is recognised as non-self and haemocytes (blood cells) aggregate around the egg, forming a multilayered capsule. Cytokines and other proteins are thought to be involved in mediating haemocyte aggregation behaviour (Strand & Pech, 1995). The subsequent deposition of melanin around the haemocyte-egg aggregate involves crystal cells (a separate class of haemocytes) and enzymes of the phenoloxidase-cascade (Strand & Pech, 1995). If deposition of melanin leads to a closed, blackened capsule, the parasitoid egg dies, possibly as a result of starvation or asphyxiation, or possibly due to toxic substances emanating from the capsule (Nappi *et al.*

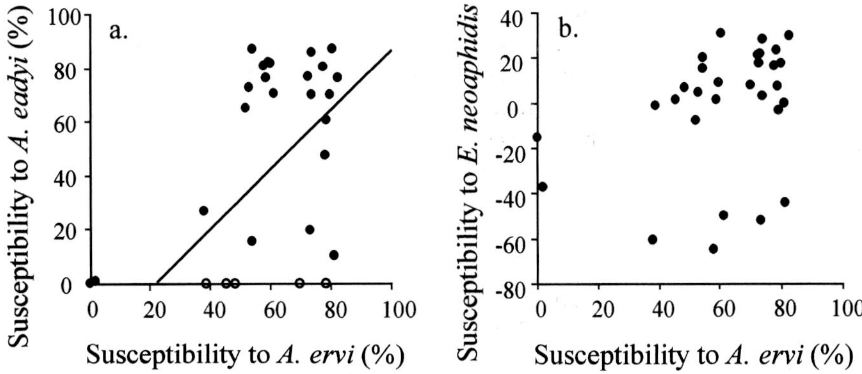

Fig. 2. Correlation amongst *Acyrthosiphon pisum* clones between susceptibility to *Aphidius ervi* and susceptibility to (a) *A. eadyi* or to (b) *Erynia neoaphidis*. The open circles in (a) are the clones that do not mummify after attack by *A. eadyi* which fail to reproduce. The susceptibility values to *E. neoaphidis* are an index. See Ferrari *et al.* (2001) for experimental details.

1995; Nappi & Vass, 1998). When the host survives, the encapsulated egg is usually visible in the abdomen as a black dot.

The parasitoid species attacking *D. melanogaster* have evolved different counter-defence mechanisms to avoid their eggs becoming encapsulated. The egg chorion of *A. tabida* has proteinaceous filaments, which cause the eggs to stick to and subsequently become hidden in host tissue, away from circulating haemocytes (Kraaijeveld & van Alphen, 1994; Eslin *et al.* 1996). In contrast to this passive counter-defence mechanism of *A. tabida*, the *Leptopilina* species actively suppress the host's immune system. Ovipositing females inject virus-like particles into the host (Rizki & Rizki, 1990; Dupas *et al.* 1996), which are believed to enter the host's haemocytes and cause apoptosis (Rizki & Rizki, 1990).

The encapsulation ability of *D. melanogaster* and the level of counter-defence of *A. tabida* shows considerable variation, both at a geographic level and within populations (reviewed in Kraaijeveld & Godfray, 1999). The evidence so far (based mostly on the interaction between *D. melanogaster* and *A. tabida*; Kraaijeveld & Godfray, 2001) does not indicate that this variation can be explained by local adaptation (where hosts are better adapted to sympatric than to allopatric parasitoids or vice versa; see Kaltz & Shykoff, 1998, for a review of local adaptation in host-parasite systems). There is also no evidence that specific genotypes of the host are resistant to specific genotypes of the parasitoid. Rather, it seems that both defence of *D. melanogaster* and counter-defence of *A. tabida* are traits analogous to the running speeds of a predator and its prey. The *relative* resistance of different host populations appears to be independent of the parasitoid population attacking them and, similarly, the *relative* counter-resistance of different parasitoid populations is independent of which host population they parasitise. Genotype-specificity might play a role, however, in the interaction between *D. melanogaster* and *L. boulardi*, as there is some evidence that *L. boulardi* survives better in sympatric than in allopatric host populations (Carton, 1984; but see Kraaijeveld *et al.* 1998).

The pupae of *D. melanogaster* are attacked by a small number of parasitoid species, of which the pteromalid, *Pachycrepoideus vindemiae*, is the commonest in Europe (Carton *et al.* 1986). *P. vindemiae* lays its eggs in the space between the actual pupa and the puparium. As such, it is an ectoparasitoid and its eggs do not come into contact with the host's immune system. However, the parasitoid has to drill through the puparial wall to lay its eggs. As in the house fly example mentioned above, the puparial wall is the main defence barrier of *D. melanogaster* pupae against pupal parasitoids.

Costs of actual defence

Oviposition of a parasitoid egg into a *D. melanogaster* larva leads to an increase in the number of circulating haemocytes, followed by the production of a melanised capsule (Carton & Kitano, 1979; Nappi, Carton & Frey, 1991). Whether capsule formation is successful or not, these activities are likely to require resources.

Carton & David (1983) showed that successful encapsulation of *L. boulardi* eggs by *D. melanogaster* leads to smaller adult flies and reduced female fecundity. Encapsulation of *A. tabida* eggs also results in a reduction of adult size and lower fecundity in females (Fellowes, Kraaijeveld & Godfray, 1999*a*). This study also looked at the costs of actual defence against *A. tabida* in males. When only given the opportunity to mate once, males which had successfully encapsulated a parasitoid egg obtained less offspring from this single mating than males which had not been parasitised. However, no difference was found when males were allowed to mate more than once with females. Hoang (2001) showed that flies which had successfully encapsulated an egg of *A. tabida* had reduced resistance to desiccation and starvation. Flies surviving parasitism lived 12% shorter than unparasitised control flies when they were maintained under desiccating conditions and 14% shorter when deprived of food. As stress resistance is correlated with body size in *D. melanogaster* (Djawdan *et al.* 1998), the decreased resistance to desiccation and starvation is likely to be an additional consequence of the reduction in body size of flies surviving parasitism.

Activation of the immune system after parasitism by *A. tabida*, whether successful in encapsulating the parasitoid egg or not, results in a reduction in larval feeding rate (Tiën *et al.* 2001). Feeding rate, the frequency of retractions of the cephalopharyngeal skeleton, is an important determinant of larval competitive ability (Joshi & Mueller, 1988, 1996). The reduction in feeding rate in *D. melanogaster* larvae after parasitism may result in parasitised larvae having a lower competitive ability than unparasitised larvae. We found no reduction in feeding rate when *D. subobscura* larvae were parasitised by *A. tabida* (Tiën *et al.* 2001). *D. subobscura* is one of the most common *Drosophila* species on fermenting fruits and has no immune response against parasitoids (Kraaijeveld & van der Wel, 1994). The lack of a reduction in feeding rate in parasitised larvae of this species indicates that parasitism *per se* does not reduce feeding rate. This observation increases the likelihood that the reduction of feeding rate in *D. melanogaster* after parasitism reflects a cost of actual defence.

A further indication that defence requires limiting resources comes from the observation that the probability of encapsulation of *L. boulardi* eggs by *D. melanogaster* larvae decreases with larval crowding (Wajnberg *et al.* 1990). A major consequence of crowding is increased competition for food amongst the larvae, and reduced food intake may mean less resources available for defence. However, an alternative explanation is that the increased build-up of waste products in crowded conditions harms the larvae and has a negative effect on their immune system. Encapsulation was not reduced in crowded larvae parasitised by *A. tabida* or *L. heterotoma* (Tiën *et al.* 2001). Whether this reflects a difference between the immune responses to *L. boulardi* and the other two species, or simply a difference in the design of the experiment, is not clear.

Apart from encapsulation, the phenoloxidase cascade is also involved in puparium formation and melanin-precursors are incorporated into the hardening puparial wall (Fraenkel & Rudall, 1947). We may therefore expect activation of the immune system to have an effect on puparium formation: resources used up by the immune system cannot be used again for puparium formation. Indeed, puparia of larvae which have successfully encapsulated *A. tabida* eggs have thinner walls than those of unparasitised larvae (Fellowes *et al.* 1998*b*). A thinner puparial wall is likely to lead to greater vulnerability to physical damage or desiccation, and also to increased susceptibility to the pupal parasitoid, *P. vindemiae* (Fellowes *et al.* 1998*b*).

Female flies can potentially detect whether a male has successfully encapsulated a parasitoid egg, as the capsule is visible through the abdominal wall. Should she discriminate between capsule-bearing and unparasitised males? On the one hand, capsule-bearing male flies advertise having genes for resistance against parasitoids, which would make them more attractive as mates. On the other hand, males with a capsule also advertise the fact that they failed to avoid parasitism in the first place, and they have reduced insemination capabilities (see above), which would make them less attractive mates. These two alternative predictions were tested in experiments where virgin females were released in cages with equal numbers of capsule-bearing and unparasitised males. Matings with both types of males occurred with equal frequencies, and hence there is no evidence that female flies choose for or against capsule-bearing male flies (Kraaijeveld, Emmett & Godfray, 1997).

Costs of standing defences

In order to measure the costs of standing defences, we selected replicate lines of *D. melanogaster* for increased resistance to *A. tabida* and, in a separate experiment, to *L. boulardi*. In five generations, encapsulation ability increased from 5% to 60% in the experiments with *A. tabida*, and from 0·5% to 45% in the experiments with *L. boulardi* (Kraaijeveld & Godfray, 1997; Fellowes, Kraaijeveld & Godfray, 1998*a*). We measured total haemocyte numbers in the *A. tabida*-selected lines and their controls and found that the increased resistance to *A. tabida* is associated with a doubling of the number of circulating haemocytes (Kraaijeveld, Limentani & Godfray, 2001*b*). This is consistent with the positive correlation that Eslin & Prévost (1998) found across species when they measured encapsulation ability and haemocyte numbers in *D. melanogaster* and five related species. Preliminary results (unpublished data) show no increase in phenoloxidase activity in the selected lines.

We tested whether there was a cost of standing defence by comparing selected and control lines for a number of life-history traits, ranging from egg viability to female fecundity (Kraaijeveld & Godfray, 1997). When flies were reared with excess larval food, we found no difference between control and selection lines in any of these traits. This was not unexpected as trade-offs are more likely to become manifest when organisms are stressed (Stearns, 1992; Bergelson & Purrington, 1996). As competition for food between larvae is important in natural *Drosophila* populations (Atkinson, 1979), we varied the level of larval competition and compared

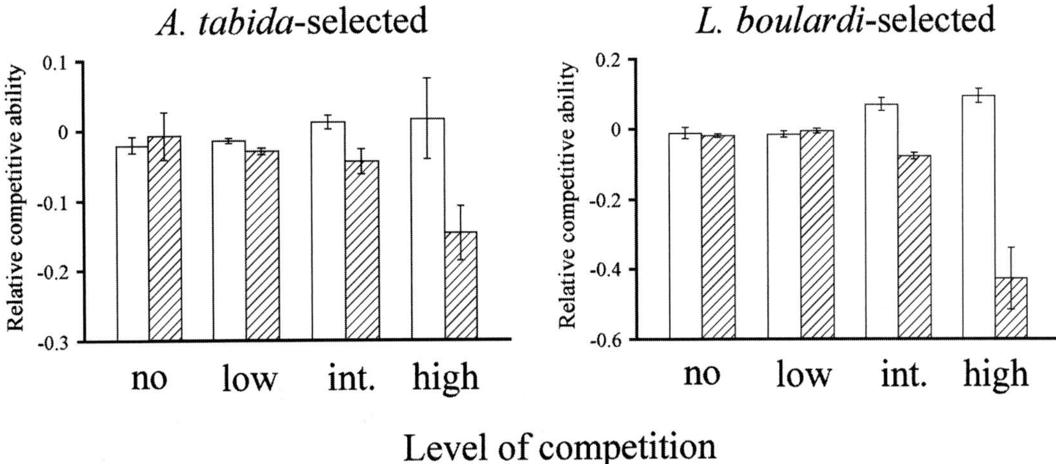

Fig. 3. Competitive ability (relative to a reference strain of fly) at different levels of larval competition of *Drosophila melanogaster* lines selected for resistance against parasitoids (hatched bars) and their respective control lines (white bars). Left panel shows results of selection experiments using *Asobara tabida*; right panel shows results using *Leptopilina boulardi*. Each bar is mean of four replicate lines ± S.E.; competitive ability is calculated as $\ln(e/(r+1))$, where e is the number of surviving experimental (control or selection) flies and r the number of surviving reference flies; 'no', 'low', 'int' and 'high' levels of competition refer to 30 larvae on, respectively, 0·4, 0·2, 0·1 and 0·05 ml of a yeast suspension. See Kraaijeveld & Godfray (1997) for experimental details.

control and selection lines. Fixed numbers of larvae from either control or selection lines were placed on food patches of varying size together with a fixed number of larvae from a standard reference strain (in our case an eye-colour mutant). Fig. 3 shows the main result: at higher levels of competition, larvae from both the lines selected for resistance against *A. tabida* and against *L. boulardi* showed a reduced relative competitive ability compared to larvae from their respective control lines (Kraaijeveld & Godfray, 1997; Fellowes *et al.* 1998*a*). We found no significant differences between individuals from control and selection lines in development time, adult size or fluctuating asymmetry.

As mentioned above, larval feeding rate is an important determinant of competitive ability. We measured feeding rates of larvae from the control and selection lines and found that the reduction in competitive ability of the lines selected for high resistance is associated with a decrease in larval feeding rate (Fellowes, Kraaijeveld & Godfray, 1999*b*). There were no differences between pupae from control and selection lines in fat reserves (measured by ether extraction; unpublished data). The difference in feeding rate between larvae from selected and control lines was much greater than that found between parasitised and unparasitised larvae from the same population (see above). To investigate further the trade-off between resistance and competitive ability, we are currently conducting replicated experiments in which larvae from a population with high resistance are reared in crowded and uncrowded conditions (A. Sanders, unpublished). If the trade-off between resistance and competitive ability is direct and symmetrical, it is expected that resistance will decrease in the crowded lines.

The reason for the negative association between haemocyte number and feeding rate is not clear at the moment. One possibility is that there is a switch in the general energy budget of a larva away from investment in a trophic function to investment in the immune system. An alternative, more specific, explanation involves the early development of the larva: the head musculature and the haemopoietic organ (where haemocytes are produced) both originate from the same part of the embryo (Fullilove, Jacobson & Turner, 1977; Tepass *et al.* 1994). Increased allocation of tissue to the future haemopoietic organ may be at the expense of future muscle tissue. A third potential explanation (suggested to us by M. Siva-Jothy) is that a doubling of the number of circulating haemocytes increases the viscosity of the haemolymph, leading to lower rates of resource supply (such as glucose) to working muscles.

Given that parasitoid species use a variety of counter-defence mechanisms, trade-offs between resistance to different parasitoid species might occur. We found no evidence for this kind of trade-off, however. Selection for increased resistance to *A. tabida* and *L. boulardi* both lead to increased resistance to *L. heterotoma* (Fellowes, Kraaijeveld & Godfray, 1999*c*). This is consistent with positive correlations that have been found amongst isofemale lines for resistance against *L. boulardi* and *L. heterotoma* (Boulétreau & Wajnberg, 1986; Delpuech, Frey & Carton, 1994).

Cross-resistance is not necessarily symmetric (Fig. 4): selection for increased resistance to *A. tabida* leads to a very small, non-significant increase in resistance to *L. boulardi* (left panel of Fig. 4). In contrast, lines selected for increased resistance to *L. boulardi* are as resistant against *A. tabida* as the lines

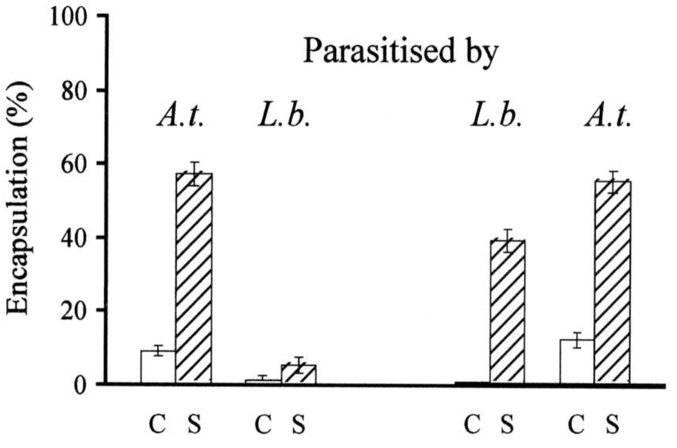

Fig. 4. Cross-resistance (measured by percentage encapsulation) by *Drosophila melanogaster* lines selected for resistance against either *Asobara tabida* or *Leptopilina boulardi* (S, hatched bars) and their respective control lines (C, white bars). Left panel shows results of selection experiments using *A. tabida*; right panel shows results using *L. boulardi*. Within each panel, the left pair of bars shows encapsulation of the parasitoid species used in the selection experiment itself (*A.t.* in the case of the *A. tabida*-selected lines, *L.b.* in the case of the *L. boulardi*-selected lines), the right pair of bars shows encapsulation of the other parasitoid species. Each bar is mean of four replicate lines ± S.E. See Fellowes *et al.* (1999*c*) for experimental details.

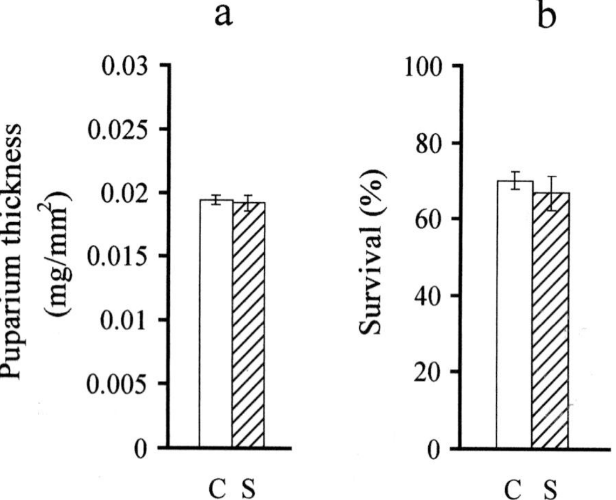

Fig. 5. (a) Puparium thickness (determined by dividing the weight of empty puparia by their surface area, assuming puparia to be ellipsoid) of *Drosophila melanogaster* lines selected for resistance against *Asobara tabida* (S, hatched bar) and control lines (C, white bar). Each bar shows mean of four replicate lines ± S.E. See Green (2000) for experimental details. (b) Survival of *Drosophila melanogaster* lines selected for resistance against *Asobara tabida* (S, hatched bar) and control lines (C, white bar) after exposure of pupae to *Pachycrepoideus vindemiae*. Each bar shows mean of four replicate lines ± S.E. See Green (2000) for experimental details.

that were actually selected for resistance against that species (right panel of Fig. 4; Fellowes *et al.* 1999*c*). This suggests that the immune system of *D. melanogaster* has two components: a general component, effective against parasitoids in general, and a specific component, required in addition for resistance against the more specialised parasitoid *L. boulardi*.

As mentioned above, encapsulation and puparium formation share a common pool of resources. Therefore, selection for increased encapsulation ability could have an effect on puparium formation and thus on resistance to pupal parasitoids. However, Green (2000) found no difference in the thickness of the puparial wall of the lines selected for increased resistance against *A. tabida* and their controls (Fig. 5*a*). He also directly examined the susceptibility of the two classes of hosts to parasitoid attack by offering females of the pupal parasitoid *P. vindemiae* a choice between pupae from the control and selection lines. Survival of flies after exposure to parasitoids did not differ between control and selection lines (Fig. 5*b*), confirming equal susceptibility. These results are consistent with the lack of correlation amongst isofemale lines for resistance to larval and pupal parasitoids (Delpuech *et al.* 1994).

CONCLUSION

Studies on a range of insect-parasite interactions have shown that resistance to parasites has costs. These costs can be associated with maintaining the machinery of an immune system and/or actually using it. Details of the nature and magnitude of these costs vary from system to system. Different life stages may also differ in the costs of resistance they experience. In *D. melanogaster* resistance against parasitoids, the costs of maintenance are mainly expressed in the larva (reduced competitive ability), whereas the costs of actual defence are most apparent in the adult (reduced size and fecundity) and pupa (thinner puparial wall and increased susceptibility to pupal parasitoids), and to a lesser extent in the larva (possibly reduced competitive ability).

In none of the insect-parasite systems studied so far have trade-offs been found between resistance to different natural enemies, such as found in the snail *Lymnaea stagnalis* (Rigby & Jokela, 2000): correlations were either positive or absent. In both insect-parasitoid systems we have studied, a high level of resistance against one parasitoid species does not necessarily guarantee a high level of resistance against the other. Interestingly, in *D. melanogaster*, it was the more specialist parasitoid that appeared harder to evolve resistance to, while with the pea aphid fewer clones were resistant to the more generalist species. So far the available evidence from insect-parasitoid systems suggests resistance and counter-resistance are graded traits without local interactions between host and parasitoid genotypes. This question has been little studied in insect-parasitoid interactions, though specificity at a genetic level in resistance against parasites has been found in, for instance, snails (Lively, 1999) and *Daphnia* (Carius, Little & Ebert, 2001).

Higher resistance in the host will lead to selection for increased levels of counter-defence in the parasite. Like defence, counter-defence may be costly. Very few studies have looked at this aspect of the reciprocal evolution of defence and counter-defence. In the bacteriophage T7, adaptation to a resistant strain of the bacterium *E. coli* led to reduced competitive ability (Chao, Levin & Stewart, 1977). In *A. tabida*, selection for increased ability to prevent encapsulation by *D. melanogaster* resulted in the parasitoid eggs becoming more embedded in host tissue, away from circulating haemocytes. Eggs of parasitoids from the selection lines hatched, on average, two and a half hours later than those of the control lines (Kraaijeveld *et al.* 2001*a*), presumably a result of lower rates of nutrients and oxygen reaching the embryo in the embedded egg. The delay in egg hatching may disadvantage the parasitoid larva if it has to compete for the host with other parasitoid larvae, of the same or a different species.

Although more studies are needed to confirm its generality, a tentative conclusion that emerges from insect-parasite systems is that costs of resistance only become apparent in situations of resource limitation, as has been found more commonly in plants (Bazzaz *et al.* 1987; Herms & Mattson, 1992; Bergelson & Purrington, 1996). The extent of competition for resources will often be linked to population density. Thus, density-dependent costs of defence and counter-defence directly link population dynamics and evolutionary dynamics (Hochberg & Holt, 1995; Doebeli, 1997; Sasaki & Godfray, 1999; Fellowes & Travis, 2000). Costs of defence and counter-defence are likely to play to pivotal role in the interaction between organisms and their natural enemies.

ACKNOWLEDGEMENTS

We are grateful to Mark Fellowes, Pete Futerman, Darren Green, Jens Rolff, Amy Sanders and Mike Siva-Jothy for valuable discussion.

REFERENCES

ATKINSON, W. D. (1979). A field investigation of larval competition in domestic *Drosophila*. *Journal of Animal Ecology* **48**, 91–102.

BARNES, A. I. & SIVA-JOTHY, M. T. (2000). Density-dependent prophylaxis in the mealworm beetle *Tenebrio molitor* L. (Coleoptera: Tenebrionidae): cuticular melanization is an indicator of investment in immunity. *Proceedings of the Royal Society London B* **267**, 177–182.

BAZZAZ, F. A., CHIARIELLO, N. R., COLEY, P. D. & PITELKA, L. F. (1987). Allocating resources to reproduction and defense. *BioScience* **37**, 58–67.

BERGELSON, J. & PURRINGTON, C. B. (1996). Surveying patterns in the cost of resistance in plants. *American Naturalist* **148**, 536–558.

BOOTS, M. & BEGON, M. (1993). Trade-offs with resistance to a granulosis virus in the Indian meal moth, examined by a laboratory evolution experiment. *Functional Ecology* **7**, 528–534.

BOULÉTREAU, M. & WAJNBERG, E. (1986). Comparative responses of two sympatric parasitoid cynipids to the genetic and epigenetic variations of the larvae of their host, *Drosophila melanogaster*. *Entomologia Experimentalis et Applicata* **41**, 107–114.

CARIUS, H. J., LITTLE, T. J. & EBERT, D. (2001). Genetic variation in a host-parasite association: potential for coevolution and frequency-dependent selection. *Evolution* **55**, 1136–1145.

CARTON, Y. (1984). Analyse expérimentale de trois niveaux d'interaction entre *Drosophila melanogaster* et le parasite *Leptopilina boulardi* (sympatrie, allopatrie, xénopatrie). *Génétique, Sélection, Evolution* **16**, 417–430.

CARTON, Y., BOULÉTREAU, M., VAN ALPHEN, J. J. M. & VAN LENTEREN, J. C. (1986). The *Drosophila* parasitic wasps. In *The Genetics and Biology of Drosophila*. **Volume 3e** (ed. Ashburner, M., Carson, L. & Thompson, J. N.), pp. 347–394. London, Academic Press..

CARTON, Y. & DAVID, J. R. (1983). Reduction of fitness in *Drosophila* adults surviving parasitization by a cynipid wasp. *Experientia* **39**, 231–233.

CARTON, Y. & KITANO, H. (1979). Changes in the hemocyte population of *Drosophila* larvae after single and multiple parasitization by *Cothonaspis* (parasitic Cynipidae). *Journal of Invertebrate Pathology* **34**, 88–89.

CHAO, L., LEVIN, B. R. & STEWART, F. M. (1977). A complex community in a simple habitat: experimental study with bacteria and phage. *Ecology* **58**, 369–378.

DE GREGORIO, E., SPELLMAN, P. T., RUBIN, G. M. & LEMAITRE, B. (2001). Genome-wide analysis of the *Drosophila* immune response by using oligonucleotide microarrays. *Proceedings of the National Academy of Sciences, USA* **98**, 12590–12595.

DELPUECH, J. M., FREY, E. & CARTON, Y. (1994). Genetic and epigenetic variation in suitability of a *Drosophila* host to three parasitoid species. *Canadian Journal of Zoology* **72**, 1940–1944.

DJAWDAN, M., CHIPPINDALE, A. K., ROSE, M. R. & BRADLEY, T. J. (1998). Metabolic reserves and evolved stress resistance in *Drosophila melanogaster*. *Physiological Zoology* **71**, 584–594.

DOEBELI, M. (1997). Genetic variation and the persistence of predator-prey interactions in the Nicholson-Bailey model. *Journal of Theoretical Biology* **188**, 109–120.

DOUMS, C. & SCHMID-HEMPEL, P. (2000). Immunocompetence in workers of a social insect, *Bombus terrestris* L., in relation to foraging activity and parasitic infection. *Canadian Journal of Zoology* **78**, 1060–1066.

DUPAS, S., BREHÉLIN, M., FREY, D. F. & CARTON, Y. (1996). Immune suppressive virus-like particles in a *Drosophila*-parasitoid: significance of their intraspecific morphological variations. *Parasitology* **113**, 207–212.

ESLIN, P., GIORDANENGO, P., FOURDRAIN, Y. & PRÉVOST, G.

(1996). Avoidance of encapsulation in the absence of VLP by a braconid parasitoid of *Drosophila* larvae: an ultrastructural study. *Canadian Journal of Zoology* **74**, 2193–2198.

ESLIN, P. & PRÉVOST, G. (1998). Haemocyte load and immune resistance to *Asobara tabida* are correlated in species of the *Drosophila melanogaster* subgroup. *Journal of Insect Physiology* **44**, 807–816.

FELLOWES, M. D. E., KRAAIJEVELD, A. R. & GODFRAY, H. C. J. (1998*a*). Trade-off associated with selection for increased ability to resist parasitoid attack in *Drosophila melanogaster*. *Proceedings of the Royal Society London B* **265**, 1553–1558.

FELLOWES, M. D. E., KRAAIJEVELD, A. R. & GODFRAY, H. C. J. (1999*a*). The relative fitness of *Drosophila melanogaster* (Diptera, Drosophilidae) that have successfully defended themselves against the parasitoid *Asobara tabida* (Hymenoptera, Braconidae). *Journal of Evolutionary Biology* **12**, 123–128.

FELLOWES, M. D. E., KRAAIJEVELD, A. R. & GODFRAY, H. C. J. (1998*b*). Association between feeding rate and defence against parasitoids in *Drosophila melanogaster*. *Evolution* **53**, 1302–1305.

FELLOWES, M. D. E., KRAAIJEVELD, A. R. & GODFRAY, H. C. J. (1999*c*). Cross-resistance following artificial selection for increased defence against parasitoids in *Drosophila melanogaster*. *Evolution* **53**, 966–972.

FELLOWES, M. D. E., MASNATTA, P., KRAAIJEVELD, A. R. & GODFRAY, H. C. J. (1998*b*). Pupal parasitoid attack influences the relative fitness of *Drosophila* that have encapsulated larval parasitoids. *Ecological Entomology* **23**, 281–284.

FELLOWES, M. D. E. & TRAVIS, J. M. J. (2000). Linking the coevolutionary and population dynamics of host-parasitoid interactions. *Population Ecology* **42**, 195–203.

FERDIG, M. T., BEERNTSEN, B. T., SPRAY, F. J., LI, J. & CHRISTENSEN, B. M. (1993). Reproductive costs associated with resistance in a mosquito-filarial worm system. *American Journal of Tropical Medicine and Hygiene* **49**, 756–762.

FERRARI, J., MÜLLER, C. B., KRAAIJEVELD, A. R. & GODFRAY, H. C. J. (2001). Clonal variation and covariation in aphid resistance to parasitoids and a pathogen. *Evolution* **55**, 1805–1814.

FRAENKEL, G. & RUDALL, K. M. (1947). The structure of insect cuticles. *Proceedings of the Royal Society London B* **134**, 111–143.

FULLILOVE, S. L., JACOBSON, A. G. & TURNER, F. R. (1977). Embryonic development: descriptive. In *The Genetics and Biology of Drosophila*. **Volume 2c** (ed. Ashburner, M. & Wright, T. R. F.), pp. 106–209. London, Academic Press.

GODFRAY, H. C. J. (1994). *Parasitoids, Behavioral and Evolutionary Ecology*. Princeton, New Jersey, Princeton University Press.

GREEN, D. M. (2000). *Coevolutionary dynamics in a parasitoid-host system*. PhD-thesis, University of London.

HARVEY, J. A., THOMPSON, D. J. & HEYES, T. J. (1996). Reciprocal influences and costs of parasitism on the development of *Corcyra cephalonica* and its endoparasitoid *Venturia canescens*. *Entomologia Experimentalis et Applicata* **81**, 39–45.

HENTER, H. J. & VIA, S. (1995). The potential for coevolution in a host-parasitoid system. 1. Genetic variation within an aphid population in susceptibility to a parasitic wasp. *Evolution* **49**, 427–438.

HERMS, D. A. & MATTSON, W. J. (1992). The dilemma of plants: to grow or defend. *Quarterly Review of Biology* **67**, 283–335.

HOANG, A. (2001). Immune response to parasitism reduces resistance of *Drosophila melanogaster* to desiccation and starvation. *Evolution* **55**, 2353–2358.

HOCHBERG, M. E. & HOLT, R. D. (1995). Refuge evolution and the population dynamics of coupled host-parasitoid associations. *Evolutionary Ecology* **9**, 633–661.

HUFBAUER, R. A. (2001). Pea aphid-parasitoid interactions: have parasitoids adapted to differential resistance? *Ecology* **82**, 717–725.

HUFBAUER, R. A. & VIA, S. (1999). Evolution of an aphid-parasitoid interaction: variation in resistance to parasitism among aphid populations specialized on different plants. *Evolution* **53**, 1435–1445.

JOSHI, A. & MUELLER, L. D. (1988). Evolution of higher feeding rate in *Drosophila* due to density-dependent natural selection. *Evolution* **42**, 1090–1093.

JOSHI, A. & MUELLER, L. D. (1996). Density-dependent natural selection in *Drosophila*: trade-offs between larval food acquisition and utilization. *Evolutionary Ecology* **10**, 463–474.

KALTZ, O. & SHYKOFF, J. A. (1998). Local adaptation in host-parasite systems. *Heredity* **81**, 361–370.

KÖNIG, C. & SCHMID-HEMPEL, P. (1995). Foraging activity and immunocompetence in workers of the bumble bee, *Bombus terrestris* L. *Proceedings of the Royal Society London B* **260**, 225–227.

KRAAIJEVELD, A. R., EMMETT, D. A. & GODFRAY, H. C. J. (1997). Absence of direct sexual selection for parasitoid encapsulation in *Drosophila melanogaster*. *Journal of Evolutionary Biology* **10**, 337–342.

KRAAIJEVELD, A. R. & GODFRAY, H. C. J. (1997). Trade-off between parasitoid resistance and larval competitive ability in *Drosophila melanogaster*. *Nature* **389**, 278–280.

KRAAIJEVELD, A. R. & GODFRAY, H. C. J. (1999). Geographic patterns in the evolution of resistance and virulence in *Drosophila* and its parasitoids. *American Naturalist* **153**, S61–S74.

KRAAIJEVELD, A. R. & GODFRAY, H. C. J. (2001). Is there local adaptation in *Drosophila*-parasitoid interactions? *Evolutionary Ecology Research* **3**, 107–116.

KRAAIJEVELD, A. R., HUTCHESON, K. A., LIMENTANI, E. C. & GODFRAY, H. C. J. (2001*a*). Costs of counterdefences to host resistance in a parasitoid of *Drosophila*. *Evolution* **55**, 1815–1821.

KRAAIJEVELD, A. R., LIMENTANI, E. C. & GODFRAY, H. C. J. (2001*b*). Basis of the trade-off between parasitoid resistance and larval competitive ability in *Drosophila melanogaster*. *Proceedings of the Royal Society London B* **268**, 259–261.

KRAAIJEVELD, A. R. & VAN ALPHEN, J. J. M. (1994). Geographical variation in resistance of the parasitoid *Asobara tabida* against encapsulation by *Drosophila melanogaster* larvae: the mechanism explored. *Physiological Entomology* **19**, 9–14.

KRAAIJEVELD, A. R., VAN ALPHEN, J. J. M. & GODFRAY, H. C. J. (1998). The coevolution of host resistance and parasitoid virulence. *Parasitology* **116** (Suppl.), S29–S45.

KRAAIJEVELD, A. R. & VAN DER WEL, N. N. (1994). Geographic variation in reproductive success of the parasitoid *Asobara tabida* in larvae of several *Drosophila* species. *Ecological Entomology* **19**, 221–229.

KURTZ, J., WIESNER, A., GÖTZ, P. & SAUER, K. P. (2000). Gender differences and individual variation in the immune system of the scorpionfly *Panorpa vulgaris* (Insecta: Mecoptera). *Developmental and Comparative Immunology* **24**, 1–12.

LACKIE, A. M. (1988*a*). Immune mechanisms in insects. *Parasitology Today* **4**, 98–105.

LACKIE, A. M. (1988*b*). Haemocyte behaviour. *Advances in Insect Physiology* **21**, 85–178.

LENSKI, R. E. (1988). Experimental studies of pleiotropy and epistasis in *Escherichia coli*. I. Variation in competitive fitness among mutants resistant to virus T4. *Evolution* **42**, 425–432.

LIVELY, C. M. (1999). Migration, virulence and the geographic mosaic of adaptation by parasites. *American Naturalist* **153**, S34–S47.

McKEAN, K. A. & NUNNEY, L. (2001). Increased sexual activity reduces male immune function in *Drosophila melanogaster*. *Proceedings of the National Academy of Sciences, USA* **98**, 7904–7909.

MILNER, R. J. (1982). On the occurrence of pea aphids, *Acyrthosiphon pisum*, resistant to isolates of the fungal pathogen *Erynia neoaphidis*. *Entomologia Experimentalis et Applicata* **32**, 23–27.

MORET, Y. & SCHMID-HEMPEL, P. (2000). Survival for immunity: the price of immune activation for bumblebee workers. *Science* **290**, 1166–1168.

MORET, Y. & SCHMID-HEMPEL, P. (2001). Immune defence in bumble-bee offspring. *Nature* **414**, 506.

MÜLLER, C. B., ADRIAANSE, I. C. T., BELSHAW, R. & GODFRAY, H. C. J. (1999). The structure of an aphid-parasitoid community. *Journal of Animal Ecology* **68**, 346–370.

NAPPI, A. (1975). Parasite encapsulation in insects. In *Invertebrate Immunity* (ed. Maramorosch, K. & Shope, R.), pp. 293–326. New York, Academic Press.

NAPPI, A. J., CARTON, Y. & FREY, F. (1991). Parasite-induced enhancement of hemolymph tyrosine activity in a selected immune reactive strain of *Drosophila melanogaster*. *Archives of Insect Biochemistry and Physiology* **18**, 159–168.

NAPPI, A. & VASS, E. (1998). Hydrogen peroxide production in immune-reactive *Drosophila melanogaster*. *Journal of Parasitology* **84**, 1150–1157.

NAPPI, A., VASS, E., FREY, F. & CARTON, Y. (1995). Superoxide anion generation in *Drosophila* during melanotic encapsulation of parasites. *European Journal of Cell Biology* **68**, 450–458.

PENER, M. & YERUSHALMI, Y. (1998). The physiology of locust phase polymorphism: an update. *Journal of Insect Physiology* **44**, 365–377.

REESON, A. F., WILSON, K., GUNN, A., HAILS, R. S. & GOULSON, D. (1998). Baculovirus resistance in the noctuid *Spodoptera exempta* is phenotypically plastic and responds to population density. *Proceedings of the Royal Society London B* **265**, 1787–1791.

REZNICK, D. (1985). Cost of reproduction: an evaluation of the empirical evidence. *Oikos* **44**, 257–267.

RIGBY, M. C. & JOKELA, J. (2000). Predator avoidance and immune defence: costs and trade-offs in snails. *Proceedings of the Royal Society London B* **267**, 171–176.

RIZKI, R. M. & RIZKI, T. M. (1990). Parasitoid virus-like particles destroy *Drosophila* cellular immunity. *Proceedings of the National Academy of Sciences, USA* **87**, 8388–8392.

RIZKI, T. M. & RIZKI, R. M. (1984). The cellular defence system of *Drosophila melanogaster*. In *Insect Ultrastructure* (ed. King, R. C. & Akai, H.), pp. 579–603. New York, Plenum Press..

RYDER, J. J. & SIVA-JOTHY, M. T. (2000). Male calling song provides a reliable signal of immune function in a cricket. *Proceedings of the Royal Society London B* **267**, 1171–1175.

SANDSTRÖM, J. (1994). High variation in host adaptation among clones of the pea aphid, *Acyrthosiphon pisum* on peas, *Pisum sativum*. *Entomologia Experimentalis et Applicata* **71**, 245–256.

SANDSTRÖM, J. & PETTERSON, J. (1994). Amino acid composition of phloem sap and the relation to interspecific variation in pea aphid (*Acyrthosiphon pisum*) performance. *Journal of Insect Physiology* **38**, 93–99.

SASAKI, A. & GODFRAY, H. C. J. (1999). A model for the coevolution of resistance and virulence in coupled host-parasitoid interactions. *Proceedings of the Royal Society London B* **266**, 455–463.

SHELDON, B. & VERHULST, S. (1996). Ecological immunity: costly parasite defences and trade-offs in evolutionary ecology. *Trends in Ecology and Evolution* **11**, 317–321.

SIVA-JOTHY, M. T. (2000). A mechanistic link between parasite resistance and expression of a sexually selected trait in a damselfly. *Proceedings of the Royal Society London B* **267**, 2523–2527.

SIVA-JOTHY, M. T., TSUBAKI, Y. & HOOPER, R. E. (1998). Decreased immune response as a proximate cost of copulation and oviposition in a damselfly. *Physiological Entomology* **23**, 274–277.

SIVA-JOTHY, M. T., TSUBAKI, Y., HOOPER, R. E. & PLAISTOW, S. J. (2001). Investment in immune function under chronic and acute immune challenge in an insect. *Physiological Entomology* **26**, 1–5.

STARÝ, P., GONZÁLEZ, D. & HALL, J. C. (1980). *Aphidius eadyi* n. sp. (Hymenoptera: Aphidiidae), a widely distributed parasitoid of the pea aphid, *Acyrtosiphon pisum* (Harris) in the Palearctic. *Entomologica Scandinavica* **11**, 473–480.

STEARNS, S. C. (1992). *The Evolution of Life Histories*. Oxford, Oxford University Press.

STRAND, M. R. & PECH, L. L. (1995). Immunological basis for compatibility in parasitoid-host relationships. *Annual Review of Entomology* **40**, 31–56.

TEPASS, U., FESSLER, L. I., AZIZ, A. & HARTENSTEIN, V. (1994). Embryonic origin of hemocytes and their relationship to cell death in *Drosophila*. *Development* **120**, 1829–1837.

TIËN, N. S. H., BOYLE, D., KRAAIJEVELD, A. R. & GODFRAY, H. C. J. (2001). Competitive ability of parasitized *Drosophila* larvae. *Evolutionary Ecology Research* **3**, 747–757.

VERHULST, S., DIELEMAN, S. J. & PARMENTIER, H. K. (1999). A trade-off between immunocompetence and sexual ornamentation in domestic fowl. *Proceedings of the National Academy of Sciences, USA* **96**, 4478–4481.

VIA, S. (1991*a*). The genetic structure of host plant adaptation in a spatial patchwork – demographic variability among reciprocally transplanted pea aphid clones. *Evolution* **45**, 827–852.

VIA, S. (1991*b*). Specialized host plant performance of pea aphid clones is not altered by experience. *Ecology* **72**, 1420–1427.

VIA, S. (1999). Reproductive isolation between sympatric races of pea aphids. I. Gene flow restriction and habitat choice. *Evolution* **53**, 1446–1457.

VIA, S., BOUCK, A. C. & SKILLMAN, S. (2000). Reproductive isolation between divergent races of pea aphids on two hosts. II. Selection against migrants and hybrids in the parental environments. *Evolution* **54**, 1626–1637.

WAJNBERG, E., BOULÉTREAU, M., PRÉVOST, G. & FOUILLET, P. (1990). Developmental relationships between *Drosophila* larvae and their endoparasitoid *Leptopilina* (Hymenoptera: Cynipidae) as affected by crowding. *Archives of Insect Biochemistry and Physiology* **13**, 239–245.

WEBSTER, J. P. & WOOLHOUSE, M. E. J. (1999). Cost of resistance: relationship between reduced fertility and increased resistance in a snail-schistosome host-parasite system. *Proceedings of the Royal Society London B* **266**, 391–396.

WILSON, K., COTTER, S. C., REESON, A. F. & PELL, J. K. (2001). Melanism and disease resistance in insects. *Ecology Letters* **4**, 637–649.

YAN, G., SEVERSON, D. W. & CHRISTENSEN, B. M. (1997). Costs and benefits of mosquito refractoriness to malaria parasites: implications for genetic variability of mosquitoes and genetic control of malaria. *Evolution* **51**, 441–450.

ZAREH, N., WESTOBY, M. & PIMENTEL, D. (1980). Evolution in a laboratory host-parasitoid system and its effects on population kinetics. *Canadian Entomologist* **112**, 1049–1106.

Subject Index

Page numbers are for the first page number only of each article. The reader may find many mentions of the topic throughout the article.